THE "CAN HAVE" DIET AND MORE!

The Easy Guide to Informed Exercise and Food Choices

Patricia M. Stein, R.D., M.S., M.A.
and
Norma J. Winn, R.D., M.S.
Illustrated by Jim Smith

NCES, Inc.
(Nutrition Counseling/Education Services)
1904 East 123rd Street
Olathe, KS 66061

The "Can Have" Diet and More!
The Easy Guide to Informed Exercise and Food Choices

An NCES, Inc. Book

Completely revised and expanded, 1987
Revised Third Edition, 1988
Revised Fourth Edition, 1990
Revised Fifth Edition, 1992
Revised and Expanded Sixth Edition, 1995

ISBN 0-9620965-1-2

All rights reserved.
Copyright© 1995 by Patricia M. Stein and Norma J. Winn
This book may not be reproduced in whole or in part, by any means, without written permission from the authors.

Inquiries, orders and catalog requests* should be sent to:

NCES, Inc.
(Nutrition Counseling/Education Services)
1904 East 123rd Street
Olathe, KS 66061

*NCES, Inc. will provide their mail order catalog free of charge. The catalog features selected books on nutrition, exercise and eating disorders. Call 1-913-782-4385 to request your catalog.

Copyright© 1981, 1987, 1988, 1990, 1992, 1995 Patricia Stein and Norma Winn. NCES, Inc, (Nutrition Counseling and Education Services), 1904 East 123rd Street, Olathe, KS 66061.

TABLE OF CONTENTS

Acknowledgements	iv
Introduction	1
Chapter One: To Diet or Not to Diet	2
Chapter Two: The Weight of the Matter	8
Chapter Three: Use 'Em or Lose 'Em	11
Chapter Four: Safety First	15
Chapter Five: Lifting Off	20
Chapter Six: Fuel for Fitness	26
Chapter Seven: Ferret Out Those Fats!	28
Chapter Eight: Foundation For Fitness	35
Chapter Nine: Ready, Set, Go!!!	40
Chapter 10: First You Say We Can And Then We Can't (Sorting Out the Conflicting Information About Controlling Blood Cholesterol)	44
Chapter 11: Salt, Salt Everywhere and Nothing Left to Eat	53
Chapter 12: Planning a Diet for People with Diabetes	56
Chapter 13: The Food Label: What's On It and How to Use It	58
Chapter 14: How to Succeed While Really Trying!	61
Chapter 15: Table of Food Values	63
Starchy Foods: Bread and Cereal Products	64
Fruits and Fruit Juices	69
Vegetables	71
Dairy Products	75
Protein Foods: Legumes, Meat, Fish, Poultry and Eggs	77
Fats, Oils and Salad Dressings	84
Desserts and Sweets	85
Miscellaneous	89
Frozen, Canned and Boxed Entrees and Meals	93
Free Foods	98
Franchise Restaurants	99
Applebee's	99
Arby's	99
Baskin-Robbins	101
Burger King	101
Captain D's	102
Church's Fried Chicken	103
Country Kitchen	104
Dairy Queen	104
Denny's	106
El Pollo Loco	109
Godfather's Pizza	110

TABLE OF CONTENTS

Hardee's	110
Jack in The Box	112
Kenny Roger's Roasters	113
KFC	114
Little Caesar's Pizza	115
Long John Silver's	115
McDonald's	117
Olive Garden	118
Popeye's Chicken and Biscuits	119
Pizza Hut	119
Quincy's	120
Rax	122
Sonic	123
Subway	123
Taco Bell	124
TCBY	125
TGI Friday	125
Wendy's	125
Chapter 16: How Do You Alter Recipes for Lower Fat Content Plus Sample Recipes	128
Appendix A: 1983 METROPOLITAN HEIGHT AND WEIGHT TABLES	138
Appendix B: SUGGESTED READINGS	139
About the Authors	140

ACKNOWLEDGMENTS

We wish to express appreciation to Gayle Lopes, R.D., L.D., of NCES, Inc., and Patricia Johnson, R.D., L.D., private practice in the Kansas City area, for their assistance in organizing the restaurant information for the FOOD VALUE TABLE. A special thanks is due Gayle for helping contact food manufacturers and restaurant franchises, for analyzing the recipes for their nutrient content, using NUTRITIONIST IV, and for her invaluable editorial assistance.

The book benefited tremendously also from the editorial assistance of Mary Howe, Ira Stein and Gerald Hay.

INTRODUCTION

THE "CAN HAVE" DIET was first written for people who wanted to lose weight by lowering calories in their diets. It included only information about the caloric content of foods. Then, our realization that calorie controlled diets almost never work for long lasting weight loss prompted several revisions over more than fifteen years of publication. In the last edition, we downplayed the use of counting calories for weight management and emphasized exercise and the Dietary Guidelines for Americans which promote increasing fiber and carbohydrate and lowering fat in the diet.

It has become increasingly apparent that "diets don't work"—at least for permanent weight control. Our previous editions have promoted healthy informed eating choices rather than just cutting calories. In spite of recent press to the contrary quoting leading medical "authorities" who urge us to keep on dieting to lose weight, we still stand by our belief that "diets don't work." When researchers can provide us with long term results that show more than 2–5 percent of people maintain respectable weight losses from dieting, then we might change our tune.

Furthermore, we're not sold on the use of drugs to control appetite. We are still waiting for long term results to show freedom from major side effects.

Why bother at all with a book called THE "CAN HAVE" DIET AND MORE!? Because we believe that some of you will opt for a healthy lifestyle. If you do, we can help you achieve this goal without resorting to a strict diet.

Who will benefit from using this book? Almost everybody, probably! But certainly anybody who is sick and tired of going on one diet after another only to regain all his/her lost weight, anybody who is interested in adopting healthy exercise and eating habits, anybody whose blood cholesterol is too high, anybody with diabetes mellitus, and anybody who needs to lower the sodium in his/her diet. Does that leave anybody out?

We will be discussing more about our reasons for not writing just another diet book in Chapter One. Beyond that, our goals are to provide you with the essential information you need to bring the exercise habit into your life and lower your percent of body fat, lower fat and increase fiber in your diet and eat according to the recommendations of the USDA Food Guide Pyramid. Also, we will give you tips about maintaining any changes you adopt into your lifestyle.

If your major interest in modifying your diet is to lower blood cholesterol or blood sugar and you are not worried about your weight, you may wish to turn directly to the chapters which relate to those situations. The food tables are present to assist all readers in making informed choices of the food they eat depending on their particular needs.

If you have been on any diet to lose weight, please start at the beginning with Chapter One. We hope you'll be glad you did.

Chapter 1

TO DIET OR NOT TO DIET?

Incidence of obesity has risen from 1/4 of the U.S. population fifteen years ago to 1/3 of the population today—that means 58 million of us. So it's a good guess many of you reading this book are starting on another quest to lose weight. You have in mind the dismal picture of past efforts to pare down to a size you believe society finds "good", only to find your weight creeping up (after a few months or years) to at least what it was before you started tinkering with it. People who go on a diet to lose weight stand a better chance of winning a lottery than of keeping off the weight they lose.

Yet, we are still bombarded with the latest "Miracle Diet" which guarantees you will lose weight permanently! Health professionals have gotten in on the act with medically supervised fasts. Unfortunately, at this writing, these very expensive and sophisticated programs do not have any better track record over time than any other diets. We would be delighted to change that statement if someone can prove us wrong.

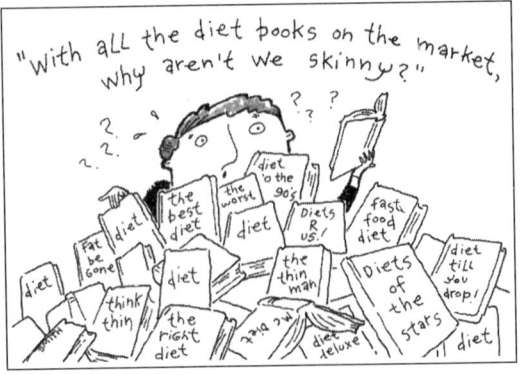

Respected professionals in the fields of weight management and eating disorders have stated that in no other medical condition is a treatment with a failure rate of 95-98 percent allowed to continue.

Susan Wooley, Ph.D., an expert in eating disorders, has posed the question, "If we don't have treatments that work, why should we use ineffective treatments?" David Garner, another expert in eating disorders concurs, "Imagine if you had a drug on the market that consistently over 20 years failed....That's what's gone on with dieting. We have 20 years of data showing that it isn't effective. We should be candid about this until there is reliable evidence to the contrary."

For treatments that don't work, we spend an enormous amount of money, approximately $32 billion in 1990. It is estimated this figure will hit at least $50 billion in 1995. When we see ads and commercials for weight loss treatments, the people pictured in them have just finished a round of dieting and have successfully lost weight as most people do on a diet. What we don't see are the results down the road when they have regained that weight and more (and, perhaps, have been on additional diets).

Questions are being raised by experts in the field about the possible long term health hazards associated with dieting and gaining, dieting and gaining. Some studies (controversial at the moment) suggest that fluctuations in body weight are implicated in increased risks of coronary heart disease and death.

We agree with the researchers who propose that all weight reducing programs should be viewed as experiments, with full disclosure that long range results may not meet your expectations.

WHAT ARE OTHER COSTS OF DIETING?

Dieting may make you fatter! What the weight loss hustlers don't tell you is that every time you go on a low calorie diet, your calorie needs go down. This is nature's way of conserving the body during a period of starvation and is how human beings have survived famines throughout the centuries. Let us give you an example of what this means to a dieter. Marie, a 41 year old inactive woman who weighed 157 pounds and was 5'2" tall, had an estimated total caloric need of approximately 2000 calories per day. Then she began a popular low carbohydrate diet of 800 calories per day. At first, her losses were impressive, and she did reach her goal weight. However, when she came to see us, she had gained back all of her losses and 10 pounds more! She claimed she could not eat over 1400 calories per day without gaining weight. Was she lying, as many health professionals think when someone makes that claim? Almost certainly not, since we now have seen that severely restricted diets can lower calorie needs by as much as 20-30 percent below pre-dieting levels. Marie's pre-diet calorie need level of 2000 per day, less 30 percent, equals 1400 calories—about the amount she claims she can eat without gaining weight.

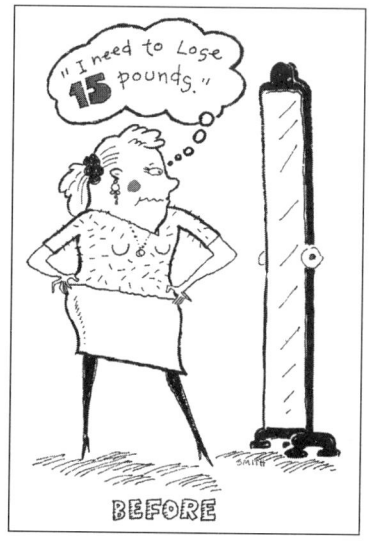

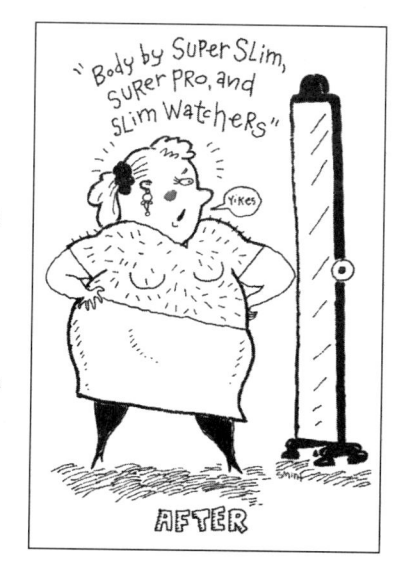

If you have experienced the "yo-yo" effect, or as some wags call this phenomenon "the rhythm method of girth control" (repeatedly losing and regaining more than you lost), you can now understand why that may have happened. After Marie lost weight on the very low calorie diet, her calorie needs were lower than when she started dieting. When she resumed more normal eating habits, she gained weight. We have known for many years that the body's response to starvation is to lower calorie needs in an attempt to preserve life as long as possible. The "problem" with our bodies is that they cannot tell the difference between dieting and starving.

Some studies have shown that with each attempt at dieting, weight loss becomes progressively slower and weight gained after dieting comes back faster.

YES, BUT I HAVE HEARD OF RECENT STUDIES WHICH SAY CALORIE NEEDS ARE NOT LOWERED WITH DIETING.

We've heard the same reports and after reading the original articles on which these reports were based, we are staying with the previous studies supported by our own clinical experience which show that dieting lowers calorie needs. Many respected authorities believe that a decrease in calorie needs is a result of a decrease in lean body mass (LBM)—mostly muscle and bone— due to aging, lack of exercise and/or dieting to lose weight. Once LBM is decreased, calorie needs are decreased and the body very efficiently stores any extra calories as fat.

Studies which claim calorie needs are not lowered with dieting were presented at an international conference on very low calorie diets (VLCDs). Some of the authors of these studies attempted to discount the impact of dieting on basal metabolic rate (BMR). Your basal metabolic rate is the number of calories you need just to sustain your body's vital functions while you are awake. This BMR accounts for most of your daily calorie needs. It is interesting to note that these reports and this conference were sponsored by companies involved in the production, distribution and sales of VLCDs to the medical doctors who use them to treat obese patients—a very lucrative business indeed.

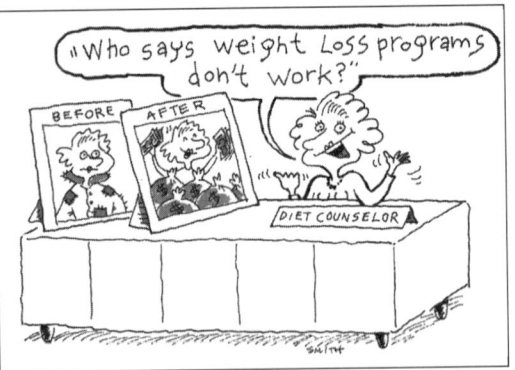

As Kelly D. Brownell, Ph.D., points out, "The issue of metabolic changes with weight cycling has not been resolved."

SO WHAT IF I DO LOSE SOME LEAN BODY MASS DURING MY DIET, WHAT'S THE BIG DEAL?

When you lose some of your muscle mass, you lose some of your calorie burning machinery. It's mainly the muscles that burn calories. And, keep in mind, your vital organs such as your heart and kidneys are part of your LBM and could be damaged. Organ failure has been reported in people who diet to extremes. If this isn't enough to scare you, consider what it means to women. Every time a woman diets without some form of exercise, she loses not only some muscle, but probably some bone mass as well. This loss undoubtedly increases her chances of developing osteoporosis (loss of bone). Also, many of these heavily promoted diets forbid her from eating the best food sources of calcium, such as low fat dairy products. For those of you who feel safe because you are taking calcium supplements, don't count on these for protection from bone problems later on. Some research shows that the food sources of calcium may be best at preventing bone problems. The increasing number of reports of young women dieting, frankly, scares us to death. A survey of San Francisco parochial schools turned up the alarming information that almost half of 9-year-old girls and almost 80 percent of 10 and 11-year-olds reported dieting to lose weight. Fifty-eight percent of the 500 girls studied considered themselves overweight, although analysis of their height and weight showed that only 17 percent were. Children and young teenagers who diet have more to lose than weight; they put their growth and development, not to mention their self-esteem, in jeopardy.

BUT, I ALWAYS FEEL SO GOOD ABOUT MYSELF WHEN I AM ON A DIET!
That may be true as long as you are doing well and losing weight. But, how do you feel when the weight starts creeping upward again, or if you find yourself in the middle of a binge? The psychological effects of bingeing and/or not maintaining weight losses are significant. To illustrate, we remember Jenni who was a world class dieter and could peel off pounds rapidly when she was on a diet. She reported an intense "high" feeling as long as her eating was under control. As soon as she got within 10-15 pounds of her "goal" weight, she would begin out of control binge eating. She felt extreme self disgust, a sense of failure, guilty, and ashamed; she could do nothing right. In short, she was extremely depressed. Does this sound familiar?

WHY DO PEOPLE ALMOST ALWAYS BINGE DURING OR RIGHT AFTER A DIET?
The debate goes on as to whether people binge for psychological or physiological reasons. It should be no surprise that a body in a state of starvation (a reducing diet) will crave food and that even well disciplined dieters will eventually succumb to this physiological need. In the 1940's, Ancel Keys, M.D., conducted a classic starvation experiment on conscientious objectors (World War II). These men were normal physically and psychologically and were placed on about one-half their normal intake of calories.

As the experiment went on, the men became obsessed with food, spent long hours planning menus and poring over cookbooks. One was found rooting through garbage cans. Several began collecting and hoarding strange items, a behavior observed in other starved animals. Some found themselves bingeing out of control and felt the same self-loathing and contempt that the bingeing dieter does. Although the men were reported to have quite tolerant dispositions before the study, they became more anxious, felt nervous and irritable with frequent outbursts of anger. They lost interest in the opposite sex and withdrew socially. In addition to being depressed, the men were found to have impaired concentration, alertness and judgment. At least two were admitted to the psychiatric ward of the hospital. Basal metabolic rate was lowered by as much as 40 percent.

When refeeding began, obsession with food and its preparation continued. Several reported bingeing. Body weight rebounded, reaching 10 percent above original levels, and body fat outdistanced original levels by 40 percent.

Many of the findings of this study parallel what happens to a dieter and help illustrate the exceptional resistance of normal individuals to weight loss. In other words, overzealous dieting (below 1200 to 1400 calories or fasting) and/or excessive exercising may lead you not only to binge, but can cause a whole host of physiological and psychological consequences. Bingeing is one way your body has of telling you that it is starving and it is time to take a breather from overly strict efforts to lose weight.

When people persist in setting unreasonable and unrealistic weight loss goals, they almost always find themselves in a vicious cycle of too strict dieting, too much exercise, binge eating, followed by feeling guilty and hating themselves. Once they are in this cycle, they are usually doomed to repeating it over and over again. If this happens to you, seek help from a health professional who is skilled in handling compulsive eating or binge eating problems. Continued dieting will only prolong your problem. In fact, almost all people who develop anorexia nervosa (self-starvation) and bulimia nervosa (severe binge eating and purging) have been on a "diet" to lose weight before developing their eating disorder.

Our bias is that the binge stems from a physiological need for an adequate nutrient intake and psychological problems are secondary. This topic deserves more discussion than this small book can provide.

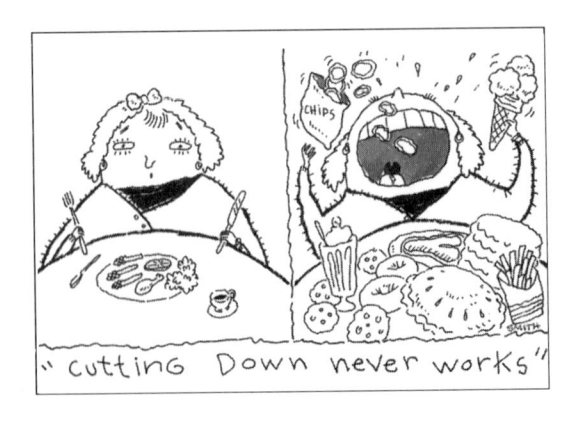

"Cutting Down never works"

CYCLE OF THE TYPICAL "DIETER"

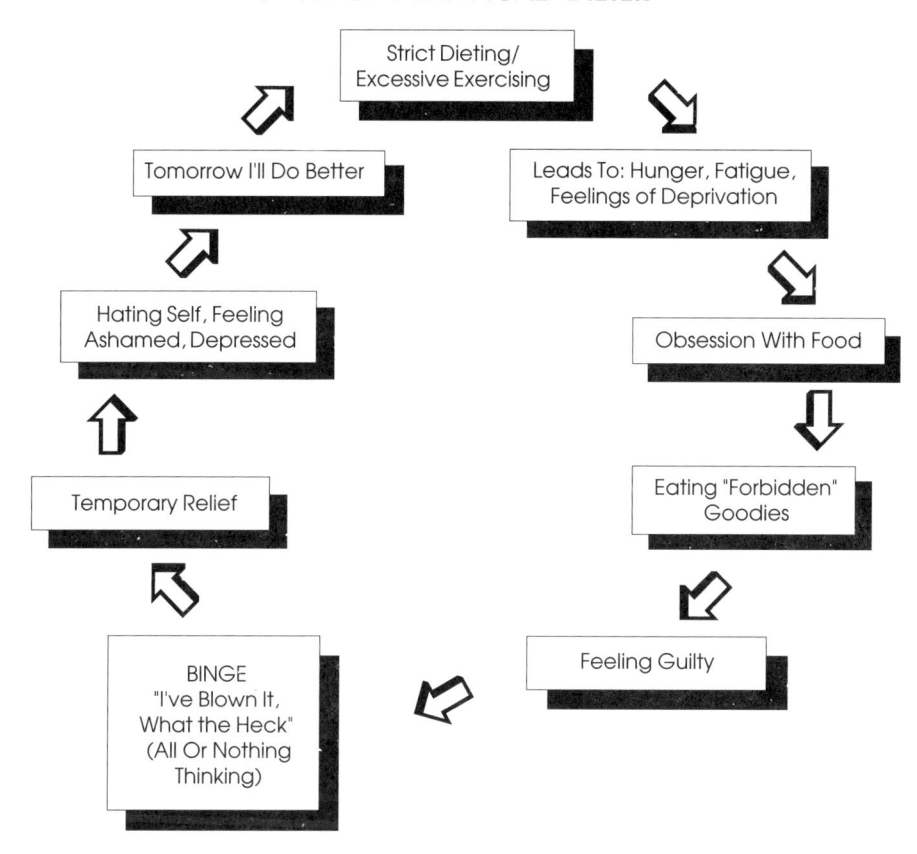

```
         Strict Dieting/
      Excessive Exercising
        ↗              ↘
Tomorrow I'll Do Better    Leads To: Hunger, Fatigue,
                            Feelings of Deprivation
   ↑                              ↓
Hating Self, Feeling         Obsession With Food
Ashamed, Depressed
   ↑                              ↓
Temporary Relief            Eating "Forbidden"
                                 Goodies
   ↖                              ↙
BINGE                        Feeling Guilty
"I've Blown It,
What the Heck"
(All Or Nothing
Thinking)
```

WHY CONTINUE READING THIS BOOK IF DIETING DOESN'T WORK?

If you have tried unsuccessfully to lose weight permanently with other diets, you will find tools which can help you lead a healthier life. They may also help you lose body fat and feel healthier when you follow our suggestions for adopting exercise and helping you learn healthier eating habits by lowering fat and increasing fiber in your diet. Read on to see how you can take these steps to better health.

IN A NUTSHELL
1. "Dieting" doesn't work for long lasting weight loss.
2. Be aware of the effect of "dieting" on the body.
3. Be aware of the effect of "dieting" on your self-esteem.
4. Be aware of the cost of "dieting" to your pocketbook. There is a bottom line. Diet programs promising quick weight loss have gained "fat" profits from the dollars of people who eventually gain only fat.
5. "Dieting" can lead to serious eating disorders such as anorexia nervosa and bulimia nervosa.

Chapter 2

THE WEIGHT OF THE MATTER

Most of you reading this book are, no doubt, reading it under the assumption you still need to lose weight. In our society, what is thought to be "fat" and what is thought to be "thin" has more to do with fashions of the "in" body style than with potential medical problems. As a matter of fact, if you trace the "in" body styles, they change quite frequently. From the rounded, voluptuous female forms of the Renaissance to the flat chests of the 1920's, to Marilyn Monroe's curves of the 1950's, to today's athletic, no fat build, you can see the ideal body style is dictated by fashion, rather than mother nature. How many of us can be "in" with our shape? Look around and note the wide variety of human forms and shapes. You can quickly see that not too many are "in" at the moment. Our advice is to make the best of the shape "Mother Nature" gave you by exercising and eating healthy.

HOW DO I GO ABOUT BEING THE BEST I CAN BE?

Aim toward a healthy level of body fat for you, usually accomplished by increasing your physical activity and eating less fat. We recommend discovering out how fat you are before you adopt major lifestyle changes.

This discovery is not as easy as looking up your weight on a chart. The standard height/weight tables are still the most commonly used methods to determine so-called "ideal" or "desirable" body weight because they are so readily available and easy to use. After debating whether to include these tables again, we decided to omit them in the body of the text. Turn to Appendix A on page 138 if you feel the urge to check out a weight range for your frame size.

Do these charts tell all? In a word, no! Unfortunately, determining degree of fatness from a standard height/weight table, even when body frame size is taken into account, can be fraught with error. Body weight is composed of lean body mass and body fluid as well as fat. The weight on the scale cannot tell you the proportion of each. But **your** healthiest weight may depend on the proportion of each.

Although the optimum level of fat probably varies from person to person, highly regarded exercise physiologists McCardle, Katch and Katch suggest the desirable level of body fat for men is 15 percent or less and 25 percent or less for women. Total body fat is not the whole story either, as it is broken down into storage fat and "essential" fat.

For men, 3 percent body fat is essential and appears to be the rock bottom level. Below this, normal physiological functioning and capacity for exercise may be impaired. The rock bottom level of essential body fat for women to maintain good health appears to be 12 percent. It is thought that the higher level of essential fat in women has to do with reproductive functions—that a woman needs a certain amount of fat in order to ovulate, conceive and carry a fetus to full term.

Although the minimum amount of total body fat (essential plus storage) for women is controversial, some experts have found that many women who fall below 17 percent body fat risk stopping their menstrual periods. Twenty-two percent fat in women is considered necessary for normal hormonal function. Furthermore, there is considerable evidence that female athletes or people with anorexia nervosa with body fat below the optimum level may develop premature osteoporosis. More study is certainly needed in this area to protect the health of women of all ages, especially dieters and competitive athletes. We are aware of the pressure placed on athletes to maintain quite low body fat percentages. Recent female Olympic athletes appeared less fat than ever, and we wonder if they are below the essential level of fat for women.

AT THE OTHER END OF THE SCALE?

What is overfat? Overfatness has been defined by some authorities as above 20 percent body fat for young men and above 30 percent for older men. The percentage for overfat young women is above 30 and for overfat older women, above 37.

How do you determine if you are over or underfat? We recommend seeking out a Registered Dietitian or other health professional who can determine your body fat percentage. The most commonly used and least expensive methods are circumference or girth measurements of selected body sites or skinfold measurements which assess fat just below the skin using skinfold calipers (skin pinchers). A combination of measurements from three or more body sites gives an estimate of body fat percentage with either of these methods. The accuracy of skinfold measurements depends on the skill and training of the person taking them. Other methods used to determine body fat percentage are less readily available and require sophisticated, expensive equipment. These are underwater weight tanks, whole body potassium counters, and electrical impedance devices, to name a few.

AM I TOO FAT?

The next table will help you determine this after you have had your body fat percentage measured.

TABLE 2-1
FAT LEVEL

	Men	Women
Too Low	**3% or less**	**17% or less**
Healthy	15% or below	22-27%
Overfat		
Young	20% or above	30% or above
Older	30% or above	37% or above

The following example illustrates how knowing percentage of body fat helped a client set realistic goals. Irene came to see us for binge eating problems and to lose weight. She weighed 187 pounds and was 5'2" tall with a large frame. Irene had been lifting weights as part of her fitness program and had a rather stocky body build. She felt terrible about her "excess" weight because according to the Height and Weight Tables in Appendix A on page 138, she should weigh between 140-159 pounds.

Her body fat percentage was estimated at 27.4 percent using skin calipers—a healthy level already, according to the chart on page 9. To get to even the highest recommended weight of 159 pounds from the Height/Weight chart, she will sacrifice some of her lean body mass. In the past, her efforts to maintain weights below 170 pounds had met with failure because her body was fighting this loss of muscle mass. Unfortunately, individuals with well developed muscle mass often are ill-advised by themselves and others when they attempt to achieve unrealistic weight goals.

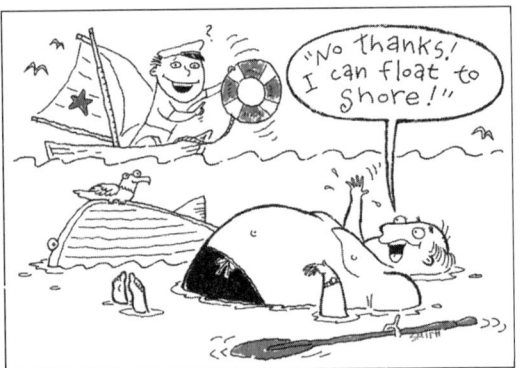

If we saw Irene today for the first time, we would simply work with her on refining her exercise program and on eating healthily. Period. End of discussion.

Binge eating is not an uncommon symptom in this situation. Irene's too rigorous, low carbohydrate, low calorie dieting efforts, coupled with her exercise program, led to frustration, guilt, and anxiety from repeated "compulsive" overeating (binge eating). When Irene adopted a diet with more carbohydrate, less fat, and more calories than she had been trying to consume, her body ceased to fight back. Her binge eating stopped and her weight even decreased. Now you can see why we strongly urge you to seek out a professional who can assess your body fat percentage and help you set reasonable, realistic goals before you undertake a weight loss program. Otherwise, you may find yourself joining the legions of unhappy dieters who are striving to achieve the impossible and end up caught in the vicious cycle of dieting and bingeing.

IN A NUTSHELL
1. Don't let fashion dictate your shape.
2. Find someone who can determine your body composition before undertaking your "Best I Can Be Program".

Chapter 3

USE 'EM OR LOSE 'EM

One of the purposes of this book is to provide the reader with assistance in choosing appropriate exercise for physical fitness and improved health. There are many "in depth" physical exercise books which we will recommend later. Our purpose, however, in the next few chapters is to provide you with a "starter kit" because we think several key points need to be made regarding exercise, fitness and health.

The old adage, "Use' em or lose 'em", certainly applies here. As we grow older and/or exercise becomes more of a spectator sport, what happens? We get a well-padded seat and well marbled muscles throughout our body. Muscle cells that are unused grow smaller while the fat cells are growing larger. When we start to move our legs and arms again (exercise), the muscle cells increase in size and fat cell size decreases. The result is an increase in our BMR, not the decrease that you will get if you diet without exercising. CAUTION! Some studies have shown that even though a person engages in exercise, if he/she goes on a very low calorie diet, metabolic rate drops anyway.

EXERCISE IS THE MEDICINE WE TAKE TO KEEP FROM TAKING MEDICINE

We used to promote aerobic activity as "the best" because of its positive impact on the cardiovascular system. Now, we're finding that strength (or resistance or weight) training has a different but just as important impact on your health. From here on, we will refer to this form of exercise as RT (Resistance Training).

WHAT'S THE DIFFERENCE BETWEEN AEROBICS AND RT?

Aerobic means air and specifically the oxygen in the air. Any exercise which moves the large muscle groups (arms and legs) consistently over a period of time increases the muscles' use of oxygen and is therefore considered aerobic. Examples are walking, bicycling, swimming, rowing, dancing, jumping rope, running in place, cross-country skiing, ice skating, roller skating and stair-stepping.

RT refers to activities that can be repeated 8 to 12 to 15 times in a row while standing or sitting in one place. Some examples are weight lifting, using small weight or resistance machines, leg lifts, water resistance exercises and rubber bands.

Recent research on a group of senior citizens has pointed up the value of RT for any age group. Not only were these seniors able to walk faster, carry heavier loads and throw away their walkers, but their activity levels increased overall with RT.

A well-rounded fitness program consists of three parts—aerobic exercise for heart and lung health, RT for strength, **and** stretching for flexibility. If

you need more reasons to choose an active lifestyle, consider the following advantages:
- Promotes heart health and helps ward off heart troubles.
- Maintains muscle strength.
- Increases your body's calorie burning rate.
- Helps ward off osteoporosis.
- Helps control diabetes and may lesson your chance of developing it.
- Increases the HDL-cholesterol, the good one, and lowers LDL-cholesterol, the bad one.
- Assists in blood pressure control.
- Reduces the pain of arthritis.
- Helps you when you're feeling blue.

WHAT EXERCISES DO YOU CHOOSE?

Some of each—aerobics, RT and stretching, but, before you choose anything, see your physician and get a green light.

Most people do best if they pick an exercise they enjoy doing. We recognize that many people who have never exercised may feel a great reluctance to even think about any form of movement, strenuous or otherwise. We also know a few of you out there, ourselves included, who say, "But, it's so bo-or-ring!" Our advice to the latter is to adopt the motto, **"Better bored than broad!"** You can choose sedentary habits and put up with a gradual loss of muscle strength and ability to carry out your daily activities, or you can choose to pursue a healthy, active lifestyle. The choice is yours!

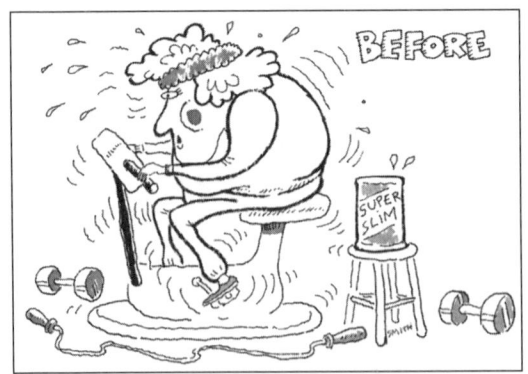

MODESTY BECOMES YOU!

In this case, we are not thinking of the type of clothing you select for your exertions, but of the size of your exercise goals. For those of you who have no recent exercise history, it is important that you set very small goals in the beginning—perhaps something as modest as walking for five minutes around your house. You can build from there.

To illustrate, let's use Carolyn as an example. Carolyn had never engaged in anything more strenuous than cooking and keeping house. In her childhood, it was considered unladylike for young girls to be sports minded. When we first saw her, she professed a strong dislike for anything connected with any extra movement. She was 62 years old, 5 feet tall, and weighed 187 pounds. In addition, she had a spinal injury which left her in constant pain and on strong pain medication.

This was Carolyn's program. Convinced of the importance of exercise in any responsible health improvement program and with her doctor's encouragement, Carolyn set as her first goal to walk for five minutes on her carpeted basement floor every other day for one week. The next week she moved up to seven minutes every other day. The third week saw her go to ten minutes every other day. To make a long story short, Carolyn was able to increase her walking gradually, up to 45 minutes four or five times each week. And she graduated from her basement to the shopping centers. As she gained muscle strength, her back pain decreased somewhat.

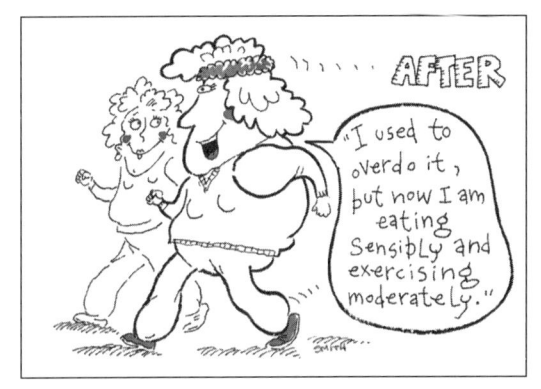

PATIENCE IS A VIRTUE.

Like most people beginning an exercise program, Carolyn expected her pounds to melt away rapidly. It took several months before she realized any weight loss. Her total loss over a six month period was five pounds, most of this occurring the last month. Her caloric intake ranged between 1200 to 1400 calories per day, according to her food records. Although we did not measure Carolyn's body fat, we are speculating that because Carolyn was so "out of shape" and had lost so much muscle tissue due to aging, previous reducing diets and inactivity, it took awhile for her to regain enough muscle mass to increase her metabolic rate.

Most people would have given up in disgust with this small weight loss. But Carolyn persevered because she was feeling so much better with her walking program and realized that her greatest hope for losing fat and feeling better was to gain muscle mass. The moral of this story is to "hang in there", even when the task seems impossible. Remember Carolyn! Many others we have worked with have surmounted what seemed impossible odds because they made a commitment and believed they could do it.

One other point is worth mentioning for those of you who expect immediate weight loss with exercising. Don't expect to lose it NOW! Be prepared for little or no weight loss at the beginning because your muscles are growing and this takes time.

Gary's case illustrates this point. Gary arrived in our office committed to doing everything right. He kept meticulous diet and exercise records from the start. Gary chose a walking program which he was able to do quite easily since he was a relatively young man without any health problems. Within a few weeks, Gary was walking 45 minutes to 1 hour a day four to five days a week. He increased his carbohydrate intake and lowered his fat intake somewhat. Gary expected to see his pounds magically melting away. However, his body weight actually increased by two pounds.

Gary was distraught until we showed him how his body composition had responded to exercising. When we measured his skin folds, we calculated he had lost about seven pounds of fat and had gained about 9 pounds of muscle mass. This gain in muscle weight accounted for the 2 pound total weight gain. Even without an actual drop in pounds, his body measurements were changing to the point that he was developing "baggy pants syndrome".

The chart below helps illustrate what happened with his body composition.

GARY'S BODY COMPOSITION CHANGE

	WEIGHT	# OF FAT	# OF LEAN
Initial	250	50	200
Later	252	43	209

As Gary exercised, his muscles "firmed up" and his body began to regain a more youthful appearance. Had he not exercised and just dieted, his weight would have been less, but his body shape would just be a smaller edition of its fatter self and not as youthful appearing. His body fat percentage might not have decreased at all, although his muscle mass would have.

Research has shown that in some cases it can take a minimum of two months before any weight loss shows up on the scales when you begin exercising as a part of your weight management program. If a person is older and out of shape, it may take even longer.

Most popular weight loss schemes promise immediate results and often brag, "No exercise is necessary!" There is no question about it, they do deliver fast weight losses, but at what expense? You have been robbed in your pocketbook, and probably of your chances for permanent weight loss. It is well known by most health professionals that this weight loss is composed primarily of water and lean body mass. We can certainly see why promoters of quick weight loss programs do not emphasize exercise as part of their approach. If they did give you the true facts, few would enroll in their programs because exercise usually slows down initial weight loss. Exercise speeds up fat loss, but also promotes an increase in LBM which weighs heavier than fat.

A word to the wise: If you stop exercising, your body fat will increase, just as it does when you stop dieting. And, when you stop both dieting and exercising as many do, watch out!

IN A NUTSHELL
1. Start with modest exercise goals.
2. Be patient.
3. Know your body composition before and during your program.

Chapter 4
SAFETY FIRST

Remember our illustration using Carolyn in Chapter Three where we stressed a modest exercise goal? Instead of trying for an Olympic Gold Medal the first time around the block, you might want to shorten the event or set a pace that's right for you. The old exercise philosophies of "No pain, no gain" and "More is better" have lost their credibility and should be buried along with all your old "diets". Current exercise practices stress "The FITT Principle": Frequency, Intensity, Time and Type. This means "how often?", "how hard?", and "how long?" do you need to exercise, as well as what type of exercise to choose.

How often do you need to exercise? Somewhere between three and five or six times per week, depending on whether you are interested in conditioning your "aerobic systems" or are using exercise as a fat loss aid. Aerobic exercising three or four times per week is usually recommended for increasing cardiovascular fitness. For fat loss, the long term goal is to exercise five or six times per week.

HOW HARD DO I EXERCISE?

This is an area of great concern. The typical exerciser shows up with more enthusiasm than knowledge about how to begin a fitness program. We have all probably experienced "the morning after" the day before when we overdid.

If you want to avoid "the morning after" or the pain of strain or possibly a worse fate, avoid exercising too hard. To discover whether you are exercising too hard, you may want to use a pulse rate chart. Some authorities suggest the "talking pace" test instead. The talking pace test means if you are too winded to carry on a limited conversation with someone while you are exercising, you are exercising at too high an intensity for you and may be doing yourself more harm than good.

If you do wish to use pulse rate to find out how hard you are exercising, here's how to take your pulse. Use your index finger to count your heart beats on the thumb side of your wrist or on the carotid artery in your neck just below your jaw. See the diagram below for the proper technique.

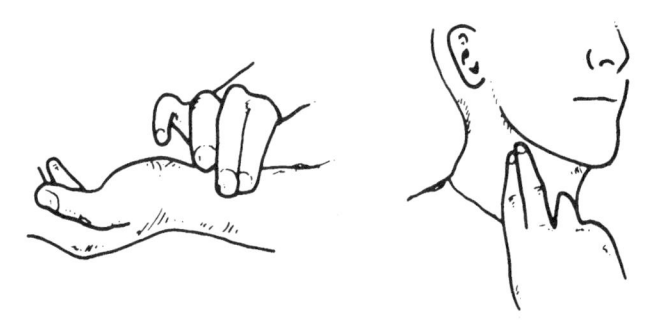

When you are just starting out, you will want to check your pulse in the middle of and perhaps several more times during your exercise session, especially if you find yourself out of breath. Practice counting your pulse for 10 second intervals (when you are not exercising) until you are able to take it easily. When you begin taking your pulse during exercise, continue the 10 second count and multiply by 6 to know how fast your heart is beating per minute. Training heart rate (THR) refers to the desirable range of heart beats per minute to obtain an aerobic training effect.

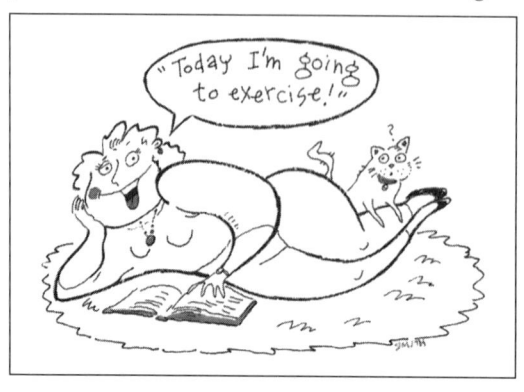

MAXIMUM HEART RATE

Unless you have had a stress test and your doctor has told you about your maximum heart rate level, you can estimate your theoretical maximum heart rate by subtracting your age from 220. To save wear and tear on your calculator and/or brain, you can consult the chart below for not only your maximum heart rate, but also the heart rates which will put you in your appropriate THR zone.

When you are just starting out, especially if you are older or out of shape, you will need to be at or below 65 percent of your maximum level.

TABLE 4-1
TRAINING HEART RATES

Age	Maximum Heart Rate	Beats Per Minute Low (65%)	High (80%)	Athlete (85%)	10-Second Pulse Count Low	High
20	200	130	160	170	23	27
25	195	127	156	166	23	26
30	190	124	152	161	22	25
35	185	120	148	157	22	25
40	180	117	144	153	21	24
45	175	114	140	149	20	23
50	170	111	136	145	20	23
55	165	107	132	140	19	22
60	160	104	128	136	19	21
65	155	98	120	132	18	20

DOES THIS TABLE APPLY TO ME?

According to Covert Bailey in his book *SMART EXERCISE*, approximately 30-40 percent of you will find your hearts beating slower or faster than the maximum heart rate, and the tables will be useless. You will need to use the "talking pace" test mentioned earlier. As a matter of fact, everyone can use the "talking pace" test. Bailey goes on to say that common sense should prevail and suggests these guidelines:

Below aerobic level	Can talk and breath easily
Doing aerobic exercise	Breathing deeply (not gasping)
	Talking haltingly (not jabbering)
In the danger zone	Wheezing (can't speak more than three words at a time)

However, for the 60% of you who have a normal heart rate response to exercise, the table can be a valuable tool to keep you from overdoing it.

Remember, "Do, but underdo!"

DO, BUT UNDERDO! is a good phrase to keep in mind here. The higher level (85 percent of your maximum) is reserved for young people and well-trained athletes. If by chance you should find your heart beating above 80 percent of your maximum, slow down, especially if you are in the danger zone of the talking pace test! You are likely harming yourself if you don't and will probably quit your exercise program within a very short period of time.

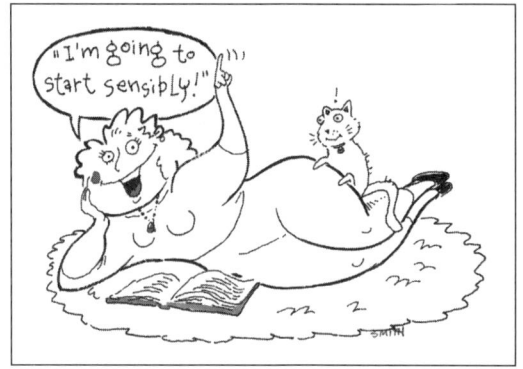

A warming up period is essential—just start off your walk or other exercise at a very slow pace and gradually increase until you are within your THR or the aerobic exercise category of the talking pace test.

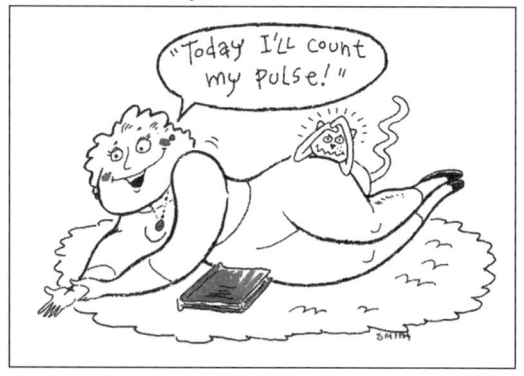

Just as important is a cooling down period when you have finished exercising. The cooling down period allows the blood to return from the lower part of your body to the central circulatory system. Otherwise, you could find yourself feeling dizzy, light-headed or worse. Slow down your pace for about five minutes to allow your heart rate to decrease. More than one person has had tragic results by not allowing themselves this "cool down" period after exercise. The case of Barbara illustrates this necessity dramatically. Barbara had just returned from an early morning jog. She jogged right into her bathroom to take a shower and turned the hot water on strong. Before she could adjust the temperature, she had passed out in the tub under the scalding water. Barbara ended up in the hospital with second degree burns over most of her body. Barbara was "lucky"—some people have keeled over with cardiac arrest. In summary, we can't stress too strongly—warm up, do, but underdo (at least at first), and cool down.

HOW MUCH TIME DO I NEED TO SPEND EXERCISING?

This will depend on your fitness level, the intensity of your exercise and type of exercise you choose. You will spend more calories when you do high intensity exercises, such as running or cross country skiing, than you will when you do lower intensity exercises, like walking or biking. The American College of Sports Medicine recommends exercising for 20-60 minutes in your THR three to five days per week for improving cardiovascular fitness. This is in addition to warming up and cooling down times.

SOUNDS LIKE I NEED TO CARRY A STOPWATCH AND PULSE METER WITH ME AT ALL TIMES!

Not to worry! If your goal is simply to improve your health, just increasing your physical activity will go a long way. If you want the benefits of cardiovascular fitness, then you might wish to approach your exercise program more scientifically. Buying a pulse meter may not be a bad idea.

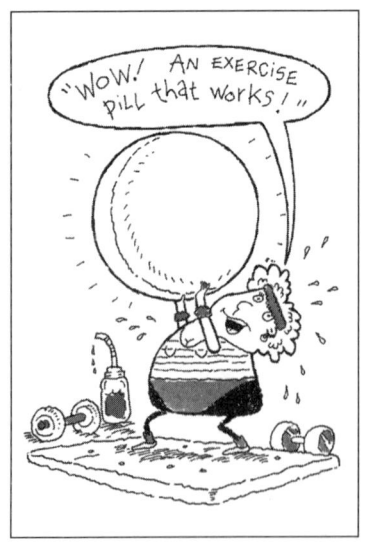

HOW LONG DOES IT TAKE ME TO GET RESULTS?

It depends on you—how fit you are to begin with. In the past, if your "exercise" has consisted mainly of "channel surfing" with your TV remote control, then you might expect to spend several months before any physical results are noticeable. You probably will feel a psychological lift after two to three weeks. If you have not been a complete couch potato, then you might see improved cardiovascular fitness, improved muscle tone and more zip in about six to eight weeks.

WHAT TYPE OF EXERCISE DO I CHOOSE?

Again, we recommend consulting your doctor. You may have some physical problems which need to be taken into account before you become the triathlete of the year. Most physicians believe walking, exercise bicycling and swimming can't be beat. Walking or cycling at a slow pace for a short period of time is safe for most people. If you have joint problems, swimming or water exercises (you don't need to know how to swim or to worry about getting your hair wet) are recommended. Pick something you can afford to do and enjoy!

We have given you a brief look at THE FITT PRINCIPLE concepts. Just a reminder—don't forget to include some stretching exercises for flexibility and some resistance training for increased muscle strength. It is beyond the scope of this book to discuss stretching and RT in detail. However, it is important to do these types of exercises correctly. For more information about how to do these exercises, we recommend reading THE WELLNESS GUIDE TO LIFELONG FITNESS from the University of California at Berkeley, published by Random House. In the next few chapters we will help you set up your exercise program and get started with it.

> **IN A NUTSHELL**
> 1. Monitor your pulse or employ the "talking pace" test.
> 2. Do, but underdo!
> 3. Warm up and cool down.

Chapter 5

LIFTING OFF!

One of the thorniest problems the beginning exerciser has is getting started. Many have wished for the magic exercise pill that requires no personal effort, but to date none has been found effective. So, you're back to relying on your own efforts. No one else can work those muscles for you.

What is this thing called "fitness"? According to the President's Council on Physical Fitness, it is defined as the ability to carry out daily tasks with vigor and alertness, without undue fatigue and with ample energy to enjoy leisure time pursuits and to meet unforeseen emergencies. To revisit the benefits of exercise, regardless of age, achieving physical fitness will improve the capacity of your heart and lungs for work, will change your body composition, will improve the flexibility, strength and endurance of your muscles and your emotional stability, not to mention your self esteem. Other benefits are that you will become more agile, have better balance and coordination, be quicker and stronger and react faster. Also recent studies indicate you will live a longer and better quality life.

THE CHOICE IS YOURS!

Now is the time for you to answer the question, "Am I willing to make a commitment to achieving this goal of becoming fit?" If you answered "yes" to this question, read on. Making this commitment means you are ready to change certain aspects of your life to accommodate some new habits of exercise. New habits of any type are not acquired just by wishing. New habits are acquired by deciding **how** the habit will benefit you, **what** you are going to do, **when** you are going to do it, **where** you are going to do it, **how** you are going to do it, and then, to actually **do** it.

WHAT ABOUT YOU?

Take a few minutes to answer the following questions about you and fitness.

1. What are your reasons for making a commitment to fitness at this time in your life? Do the costs outweigh the benefits?

The following analysis may help you decide.

FOR ME:	
Benefits of not exercising	**Benefits of exercising**
Costs of exercising	**Costs of not exercising**

What did you decide?

2. What type of exercise are you considering doing? Examine the pros and cons of each type. (Convenience, cost, special equipment needed, etc.)

3. When are you planning to work exercise into your schedule? How long do you plan to exercise at first?

4. Where are you going to do your exercise?

To help you give some preliminary thought to why, what, when and where, let's take the case of Sherry.

THE CASE OF SHERRY

Answering all of the above questions doesn't guarantee success. Sherry's situation is a case in point. Sherry considered herself a failure in her quest for fitness. She had made the choice and commitment; she knew why and she thought she knew what, where and when. Sherry was in her early fifties and believed she was overweight. During the summer, she chose fitness as a means of preventing osteoporosis and for weight management, as well as overall well-being. Her plan included a twenty minute walk, three times a week in her neighborhood after work. This plan went well until she had major surgery in the late fall. Her surgery was followed by the holiday season and a long vacation trip. When she was ready to resume her exercise in February, she had the same plan in mind. Unfortunately, this time she was unable to carry it out and didn't know why she was unable to "motivate" herself to begin again.

Many people would have quit when they thought they had failed, but Sherry was determined to form more positive health habits. In analyzing what had gone wrong with her plan, she found she was reluctant to walk by herself after dark. After she realized this was simply a "glitch" in her plan and not in herself, we were able to explore alternative courses of action that would stand a chance of success. Brainstorming for new options allowed Sherry to list several alternatives. Among the exercise options she listed were to use the stationary bicycle she had at home or to exercise with television programs. She also included videotaped exercise programs, a treadmill, a cross-country skiing device and a rowing machine. Cheaper alternatives were walking in a shopping mall or using a mini-trampoline. She considered a health club, but knew it could cost a lot.

Next, Sherry examined the pros and cons of each of her alternatives. Many fitness programs have bitten the dust because the potential exerciser did not consider the pros and cons of each alternative and made a choice that was unrealistic. The first alternative Sherry examined was whether or not to ride her stationary bicycle. Once before, she had determined that this would be her chosen mode of exercise, but had given up after a short time because the seat was too uncomfortable and the bicycle was in the basement facing a brick wall. Budding exercise enthusiasts will seldom continue a program if it is too uncomfortable or too boring. Had Sherry traded in her too small seat for a larger, more comfortable model and placed her bicycle in a room with a television set and/or reading stand, she might have enjoyed it more. Sherry built up an aversion to the bicycle and decided it would not be a realistic choice for her.

OTHER OPTIONS

Treadmills, cross-country skiing machines, rowing machines, and stair-climbing machines require a significant investment and can take up significant amounts of living space. Although Sherry did not rule out these alternatives altogether, they were not realistic for her at the time. She contemplated renting one or more of these for a trial. She rejected the mini-trampoline because she had heard an exercise physiologist discuss the risk of injuries associated with this equipment.

Health clubs require a greater expenditure of time and money than do home exercise programs. Few of us can afford the two to three hours per day commitment of time that is required for going to a health club, suiting up for exercise, exercising, showering, dressing and driving home. Sherry did not believe she had this much time to commit. Another consideration is most health clubs' dues are in the several hundred dollars per year category—about the cost of a good piece of home exercise equipment.

On the other hand, if someone needs to get out of the house, like a mom at home with small children all day, a health club can provide many positive benefits, such as socializing with other adults. Our point is that each person needs to weigh all the pros and cons based on his/her situation.

Sherry decided to purchase a low impact aerobic videotape after debating the above alternatives. She did, and reported at our next meeting that she had gotten started and had met her objective of exercising three times each week. Her plan was to continue with the aerobic videotape.

However, at the following visit, Sherry was back to thinking she had failed again. She had loaned her VCR to her daughter for a couple of weeks and had not been able to carry out her chosen plan. The problem this time was lack of a backup plan. Sherry could have gone to the shopping center and walked, even though this activity would not have been her first choice. In fact, she had taken a short walk on her lunch hour with a coworker, but had discounted this as exercise.

For an exercise program to succeed, you need to have not only Plan A, but also Plan B and perhaps Plan C. Plans B and C may not be your most favorite activities, but at least they will enable you to stay on your path to fitness when Plan A is temporarily disrupted.

GIVE YOURSELF A BREAK!

Don't think you are a failure if your plan doesn't work. All this means is that you need to go back to the drawing board and see why it didn't work and keep trying out different plans until you find one that fits you and your special needs. Sherry finally believed that she would be successful. And we agreed because she knew to take into account not only why she wanted to exercise and what exercise she was going to do, but also when and where she could get the job done consistently.

Some words you always should remember never to say are "always", "never", and "should". More new habits are trashed by a part of us rebelling and saying, "Well, I should exercise today. I said I would always exercise on Mondays and never skip a session." And, when you don't exercise every Monday, you feel guilty and say things to yourself, like "I'm a failure" or, "I've never succeeded, why should I succeed this time?" Before you know it, you have beaten up on yourself to the point that you say, "Well, I've blown it, what's the use?" A positive motto to remember here is "**PROGRESS, NOT PERFECTION**". No one we know behaves perfectly all the time. We have found our clients succeed when they make their exercise habit a choice. Once you have made a commitment to exercise, there are days when you will not feel like meeting your goal. When this happens, choose to postpone it for a day.

If you feel yourself slipping in your resolve for more than a few days, go back to your **FOR ME** analysis of the costs and benefits of exercising and see if your reasons are still worthwhile for you to continue the fitness choice. If the cost of continuing to exercise at this time in your life is too much, you can choose to stop. Perhaps you will feel like making the choice for fitness again at a later date. If your choice is to stop exercising, then it is pointless to feel guilty about it.

One more thing to consider here is that it may take six months or longer before a person becomes "hooked' on the exercise habit. Also, remember that what works for your friends and relatives may not work for you.

DO I NEED TO KEEP A DIARY OF MY EXERCISE?

We certainly recommend it! Most new habits require several weeks, if not months, of continual reinforcement to stand a chance of becoming permanent. One of the most reinforcing things you can do is to keep a record of your achievements, whether you are acquiring new exercise habits or new eating habits. If you are getting discouraged, you can look back at where you started and see how far you have come. As you begin to get more fit, your resting pulse will usually drop; this can be a very tangible measure of your progress. Take your resting pulse before you get out of bed in the morning.

GETTING STARTED

To help you get started, use the following exercise worksheet. (Make extra copies as necessary.)

EXERCISE WORKSHEET: PLAN AND DIARY

WEEK NO.: _____ DATES OF WEEK: _____ WEEKLY GOAL: _____

Day	✓ When Completed	Planned Time(s)	Activity	Exercise Heart Rate	Distance/ Duration	Comments
Monday						
Tuesday						
Wednesday						
Thursday						
Friday						
Saturday						
Sunday						

RESTING PULSE (Take Once A Week): _____

PLANNING YOUR EXERCISE:

For best results in forming an exercise habit, jot down in pencil which days and times you are planning to exercise this week. Consult your calendar to see if what you are planning is realistic and then make any necessary changes in your plan. When you follow your plan, simply make a check mark beside the completed exercise time. If you need to deviate from your plan, write down what you actually did in ink. Treat your planned exercise time as you would an appointment. Remember to mark it on your regular scheduling calendar also.

EXCEPTION TO THE RULE!

The best laid plans often go astray, including exercise plans. Vacations, illness, change of season, change in jobs and/or schedules, change in your children's schedules, visiting family or friends, change in family situations (marriage, divorce, death, income, retirement) can have an impact on your exercise schedules. When possible, plan ahead, but don't let a temporary setback get in the way of your achieving your long range goal—to be fit. Alter your plans or make new plans as soon as possible. And, if you have to stop for awhile, simply plan to resume as soon as you can. You can maintain your current level of fitness with as few as two 10-15 minute exercise periods per week. You probably won't improve, but you won't lose much ground either.

IN A NUTSHELL
1. Examine all angles, plus the costs and benefits to you before making your commitment to exercise.
2. Keeping a diary helps.
3. Making a basic plan along with backup plans is essential.

Chapter 6

FUEL FOR FITNESS

Before we go into the food section of this book, let's talk about how to fuel this fit body of yours. The fuel we get from food is in the form of carbohydrate (starches and sugars), protein (meat, fish, poultry, milk, cheese, legumes), and fat (oil, margarine, butter, salad dressings, etc.) which are our primary sources of calories. Our bodies are burning calories twenty-four hours per day. How many, at any particular time, depends on what we are doing. The more active we are, the more calories we burn. Carbohydrate and fat calories are the main sources of fuel. Protein is necessary to build and maintain our muscle mass, but can also be used for fuel if not enough of the other two sources are on hand. Any calories we don't use are stored in the body as fat.

Aerobic exercise needs glucose (blood sugar) as a starter fuel. Our bodies prepare for this by storing glucose in the liver and muscles in long chains called glycogen (a starch). When you eat carbohydrate in adequate amounts—now believed to be at least 55–60 percent of your total calories—your body will store glycogen. If you do not take in enough carbs from your food, the body is likely to get it from breaking down protein, either from your dietary protein intake or—heaven forbid—from your own body protein (muscles and organs), in order to obtain the glucose it needs for fuel. Glucose is essential for us to perform our daily activities. The brain does not function well at all without it. Some authorities compare the function of glucose in the burning of fat to the use of kindling in starting a fire. Your fire will burn better with a kindling primer, just as your fat stores will burn better if you have enough glucose to act as your "fat kindling".

WHAT IS ALL THIS ABOUT A MORE FIT BODY BEING ABLE TO STORE MORE GLUCOSE?

The more well trained your muscles are, the more glycogen (glucose) they can store. For this reason, people who train for marathons can go long periods of time on their body stores of fuel. The unfit, untrained body will "run out of gas" after a very short time because it will not have adequate stores of glycogen. Only exercise gives you well trained muscles.

WHY DO ALL THESE POPULAR REDUCING DIETS TELL ME TO EAT VERY LITTLE OR NO CARBOHYDRATE AND YOU ARE TELLING ME TO EAT A LOT?

Most veteran dieters believe carbohydrate foods are fattening. Nothing is farther from the truth. The reason these diet programs have you drop carbs from your menu is that the muscles in your body can store about a pound of glycogen. It takes almost three pounds of water to assist in the storage. Lower your glycogen stores by dropping carbs from your diet and you will experience an immediate drop in weight of several pounds. Then, when you begin to restock your muscle glycogen cupboards, you will regain this lost water weight. Your immediate thought is that carbohydrate foods are fattening. They caused you to gain weight, didn't they?

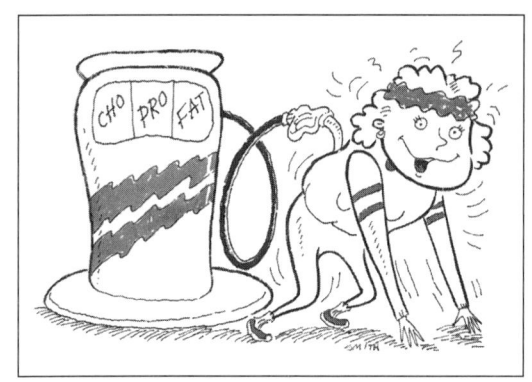

Actually, per gram, carbohydrate has 4 calories; protein, 4 calories; fat, 9 calories; and alcohol, 7 calories. One teaspoon will hold about 5 grams, so you can see that one teaspoon of sugar, a carbohydrate, has about 20 calories while a teaspoon of oil, a fat, has about 45 calories. We used to say a calorie is a calorie whatever its source, but some studies indicate that calories from fat may be more fattening than the calories from carbohydrate. It seems that as our bodies are processing our food, only 75 percent of unneeded calories from carbohydrate are converted to stored body fat, while 97 percent of unneeded fat calories are stored as body fat.

IN A NUTSHELL
1. Your body needs carbohydrate for maximum performance.
2. Carbohydrate (unless you eat more than your body needs) is not fattening!

Chapter 7

FERRET OUT THOSE FATS!

Now that you know unneeded fat calories are potentially more fattening than unneeded carbohydrate calories, are there other reasons to be concerned about the amount of fat you eat? Yes, whether or not you are lowering fat in your diet as a potential weight management tool, there are many other reasons to be interested in a reduced fat intake. Perhaps you are concerned about preventing certain health problems which have been associated with eating a high fat diet, or maybe your doctor has already prescribed a low fat diet to lower your cholesterol level. We will be discussing the use of lower fat food choices for cholesterol and for diabetes management after we finish our discussion of using a lower fat diet as a weight management tool.

If you are tired of calorie counting, lowering the amount of fat in the diet will almost automatically insure a lowered calorie intake, provided you don't get carried away with other foods.

Here's the scoop! We are going to show you an easy way to make informed healthy food choices by using fat grams.

WHERE DO I FIND THESE FAT GRAMS?

They can be found in the first column of the food tables beginning on page 64. Remember, if you keep the total fat content low in your diet, you probably will have lowered the total number of calories you are eating. Since fat is the most concentrated form of calories and one of the least visible ones, knowing the fat content of the foods you eat can help you in substantially cutting calories without the hassle of counting them.

BUT I READ RECENTLY EATING PASTA AND LOWER FAT FOODS IS MAKING US FATTER!

We read the same articles and can help you put them into perspective. It is very hard to mount a significant tally of either calories or fat if you consume more fruits and foods high in complex carbohydrates (vegetables and starchy foods), especially if they are prepared without additional fat or sugar. For example, one puny 2 ounce candy bar contains 10 fat grams and 270 calories. For the same number of calories and **no** fat grams, you can have 1 apple, 1/2 cantaloupe, and 1 whole grapefruit. The candy bar is an example of a calorie dense food with few other redeeming features. With the fruit, you not only will feel stuffed, but you will have consumed generous amounts of fiber, vitamins and minerals.

However, **any food**, even a low fat or fat free food, eaten in too large a quantity has the potential to make us fatter. If you choose to eat unlimited amounts of **any** food just because it does not contain fat, you could be kidding yourself. Exercise common sense in the matter of quantities of low fat food choices. For example, 2 cups of spaghetti (a fairly generous portion of a low fat food) with low fat red sauce has about 400 calories. If you eat 4 cups, you have doubled the calories, even though the fat content of the dish is still on the low side. Just because you are not eating much fat does not mean you are eating a low calorie diet.

The same principle applies to low or non fat foods such as candies, cookies, sugars, soft drinks and alcoholic beverages. Eating 3 low fat Oreos which contain 5 grams of fat and 140 calories is a lot different than eating the whole package just because they happen to have less fat than the original.

When you use your common sense, lower the fat in your diet and stop eating when you feel full, it **is** possible to eat a healthy lower calorie diet without counting calories.

HOW MANY FAT GRAMS ARE RECOMMENDED FOR A HEALTHY DIET?

A good rule of thumb is to aim for 35–50 or fewer fat grams per day if you are a gal and 40–60 if you are a guy. You will most likely be consuming less fat than you are now as well as a healthier diet than you were before you started watching your fat intake.

If you want to be more precise and figure your fat grams based on 20–30% of your calorie needs, as dietary guidelines suggest, then you need to know what your estimated daily calorie needs are.

HOW DO I KNOW HOW MANY CALORIES I NEED?

You won't for sure, because your calorie needs are based primarily on the amount of your lean body mass. Even though you might know the weight of your lean body mass and your body fat percent, there are no easy to use guidelines to help you figure your daily calorie needs using this information. And, your calorie needs are also affected by your physical activity level and heredity.

We have chosen to base our calorie guidelines on information presented in the 1989 edition of *RECOMMENDED DIETARY ALLOWANCES*. These guidelines are based on people engaging in very light, sedentary activities. Your own calorie needs may vary but, for the purposes of figuring your desired fat intake, these guidelines are close enough.

So, here's a table to help you in computing daily calorie needs to arrive at your daily fat intake goal. Multiply your weight in pounds by the number of calories listed next to your age range in Table 7-1.

TABLE 7-1
CALORIES PER POUND BASED ON AGE

Ages 15–18	16
Ages 19–24	14
Ages 25–50	13
Ages 51+	12

For example, Connie, who is 40 and weighs 150 pounds, has an estimated calorie need of about 1950 per day (13 x 150 = 1950). Or Max, who is 55 and weighs 175 pounds, needs approximately 2100 calories (12 x 175 = 2100).

NOW THAT I HAVE ESTIMATED MY CALORIE NEEDS, HOW DO I FIGURE 20 OR 30 PERCENT OF MY CALORIES AS FAT GRAMS?

It just so happens we have concocted an easy to use "do-it-yourself" table. See TABLE 7-2.

TABLE 7-2
DAILY LEVELS OF CALORIES AND FAT

Calories	Fat Grams (30% of Calories)	Fat Grams (20% of Calories)
1400	46	31
1500	50	33
1600	54	36
1700	56	38
1800	60	40
1900	64	42
2000	66	44
2100	70	47
2200	74	49
2300	78	51
2400	80	53
2500	84	56
2600	87	58
2700	90	60
2800	93	62
2900	97	64
3000	100	67

For example, Connie can eat 65 grams of fat daily if she aims for a fat intake of 30 percent of her estimated need of 1950 calories. If she lowers her fat intake to 20 percent of her calories, she can eat about 43 grams of fat. Our advice is for Connie (or you) to begin at the 30 percent level and, if necessary, gradually reduce your fat intake to the 20 percent level to achieve your health goals.

WHAT ABOUT COUNTING CALORIES TO LOSE WEIGHT?

We don't advise it because we have found that lowering fat in the diet is usually enough to lower fat in the body. Plus, if you don't count calories, you will avoid the physical and psychological effects of watching every bite you put in your mouth. We know, however, there are a few calorie conscious diehards out there, so we have left the calorie information in the food tables.

If you insist on counting calories, we recommend the following steps:
- Keep a diary of your current food intake for about one week.
- Analyze the calories in these foods.
- Look at the foods carefully and figure out about 250 calories a day you'll miss the least.

If you leave these 250 calories out of your regular intake, in theory you will lose about 1/2 pound of fat each week. If you start exercising regularly, this loss could amount to as much as 1 pound of fat loss per week. Notice we are talking fat loss, not necessarily weight loss, because of reasons we discussed in Chapter 3. Remember, you can avoid the whole issue of counting calories by counting fat grams or by using an even easier method described below.

YOU MEAN I CAN LOWER FAT IN MY DIET WITHOUT COUNTING GRAMS?

Some of you will do just as well making gradual changes in your diet and will be able to lower fat significantly by trying some of the "tricks" listed on the next page instead of counting each and every fat gram that goes in your mouth. You might start out by writing down the foods you currently eat for a few days and looking up the grams of fat in those foods. Then, check out some of the ideas below for trimming the fat from your food and decide what changes you are willing to make.

Bonnie, for instance, feels that looking up the foods she eats and counting fat grams is too much like all of the other times she has dieted. She did agree to write down a few day's intake, and it became apparent that just by changing from a pint of regular premium ice cream to a pint of nonfat frozen yogurt per day that she could save a significant amount of fat and therefore, calories. She liked the frozen yogurt just as well as the ice cream, so she did not feel she was making a sacrifice.

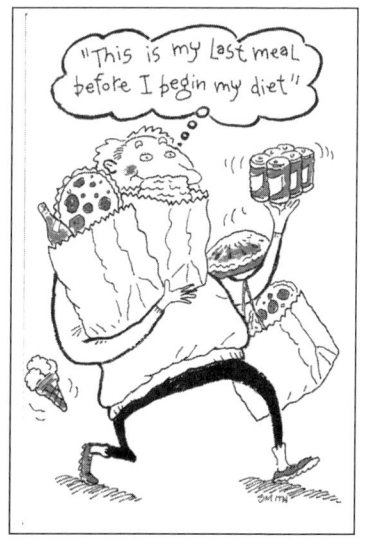

Bonnie may find other changes she can make without feeling she is giving up all that is "near and dear" to her heart.

Check out the EASY TRICKS TO LOWER FAT chart on the next page for other ideas to lower fat without having to count fat grams.

EASY TRICKS TO LOWER FAT

INSTEAD OF THIS	TRY THIS
Whole milk or 2% fat milk	1% fat milk or skim milk
4% fat cottage cheese	1-2% fat cottage cheese or nonfat
Regular cheeses	Reduced fat or no fat cheeses
Regular butter or margarine	Whipped or reduced fat margarine or nonfat margarine
Whipping cream	Reduced fat dessert topping or whipped evaporated skim milk
Cream in recipes	Evaporated skim milk
Sour cream	Nonfat plain yogurt or low or nonfat sour cream
Fats and oils used for frying	Non-stick pan sprays
Cream sauces and gravies	Thicken skim milk or fat free broth with cornstarch or other thickeners
Ice cream	Fat free frozen yogurt or fat free iced milk
Butter, margarine, salad dressings and other fat seasonings for vegetables	Spice blends, seasoned pepper, herbs, spices, lemon juice, vinegar, fat free broth, fat free cheese, reduced fat or non-fat salad dressings
Potato chips, corn chips	Pretzels, low or nonfat popcorn, fat free corn or potato chips
Regular ground beef	7-10% or less fat ground beef or frozen vegetable burgers
Regular wieners	1 gram fat wieners or fat free
Regular luncheon meats	3% or less fat luncheon meats
Beef, pork, lamb and veal	Lean, well trimmed cuts 3-4 times per week. Fish, skinless poultry and legumes more often

Check the food tables in the last half of this book for more options.

WILL IT HURT ME TO EAT ZERO FAT GRAMS?

You need some fat in your diet. Your body needs small amounts of essential fatty acids which come from the fat you eat. Your body cannot produce these fatty acids. Deficiency symptoms are scaly skin, hair loss and slow wound healing. It appears that by keeping the level of fat at 20–30 percent of your calories and including some polyunsaturated fatty acids, your diet should be adequate. See page 50 for more information about food sources.

WHAT HAPPENS IF I OVERDO? WILL I RUIN MY CHANCES FOR SUCCESS?

We suggest viewing your intake by the week instead of the day. Some days you may be under your level of fat grams and some days over. Unless the overs outweigh the unders, it will all even out. Because of this, if you run over a few grams every now and then, don't worry. If you are consistently over, analyze what is contributing to this and make plans to alter some aspect of your intake. For example, if you find that you are spending 36 of your 50 fat grams on a Big Mac and a small order of french fries, ask yourself what alternative McDonald's has that you like as well and that has fewer fat grams. Or, look at other restaurants for lower fat alternatives. Some of you may choose to brown bag your lunch to save fat grams to spend on more favorite foods for breakfast or dinner. When you use the information in the food tables to make informed choices, you can nearly always find something you like just as well or almost as well as some of the higher fat choices. Our motto has always been **"THERE ARE NO INAPPROPRIATE FOODS, THERE MAY BE INAPPROPRIATE AMOUNTS!"** Remember our other motto from the chapters on exercise because it applies here too, **"PROGRESS, NOT PERFECTION!"**

REMEMBER, USE THE TABLE OF FOOD VALUES FOR MAKING INFORMED CHOICES OF FOODS.

We have not included all this information to make your life harder. Rather, you are now in a position of being able to make your own food choices because you have the information yourself. This way, you do not need to depend on a "diet" sheet or your dietitian or doctor to tell you what you can and can't do. As long as you have decreased your fat intake overall, you should improve your chances of preventing heart disease and/or cancer. If you have diabetes, it may be better controlled.

A word to the wise! If you don't like a lower fat food, don't eat it. There are plenty of other alternatives out there that you might like.

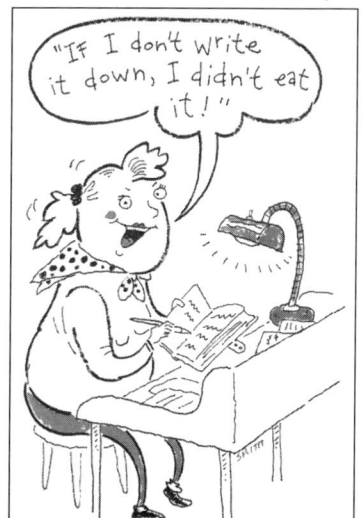

RECORD AS YOU GO!

If you're like most of us, you'll develop a severe case of amnesia regarding any foods eaten within less than 2 hours after a meal. Keeping records at the time you eat, even if it's only a simple tally of your fat grams, is a big help. A food diary helps in several ways. It can be a big awareness booster about what you are eating. More important though, a record of any new habit acts as a reinforcer in the establishment of that habit, whether it is an exercise or an eating habit or any other habit you are trying to cultivate. Also, we have found that a diary can help absolve some of the guilt feelings people have about consuming too much of certain types of foods. When you have a diary, you can look back at it and see that you have in fact not overeaten, even though you felt you had. We recommend using a small pocket notebook for your diary.

SOMETIMES MY WEIGHT GOES UP FOR NO GOOD REASON AND IT CAUSES ME TO FEEL LIKE "WHAT'S THE USE, NOTHING WORKS!"

Many times people give up when they are doing everything right and still do not get the reward (weight loss, or at least not a weight gain) they feel they deserve for all the effort they have put into their habit changes. Sometimes it pays to "play detective". Inspect your medicine closet. Some medicines you take may cause you to have extra fluid weight. Ask your dietitian or doctor about any medicines you are taking. In fact, some medicines cause an increase in appetite and eating with a resultant weight gain. It pays to know the effect of any medicine on weight.

Even a meal with a high salt content can result in a temporary fluid increase of three or four or more pounds. And, speaking of water weight—gals, don't push the panic button if you gain a few pounds of fluid close to your menstrual period or at the time you ovulate. We have observed some weight gains as high as eight or more pounds in premenstrual women which drop quickly once their period is over. It is not uncommon for even the most slim person to feel fat at the time of her menstrual period. It is not uncommon either for most women to have an increased appetite before their menstrual period begins. It may help your morale to keep a graph of your weight changes so you can predict when these periodic increases in weight will occur.

Weigh only once a week and remember, if you are exercising regularly, the scale will not show your progress immediately. See Chapter 3 again.

IN A NUTSHELL
1. Find out how many fat grams are healthy for you to eat in a day.
2. Count fat grams instead of calories to lower your body fat.
3. Use the EASY TRICKS TO LOWER FAT if you want **really** easy ways to lower fat in your diet.
4. Keep a log of your fat intake.

Chapter 8

FOUNDATION FOR FITNESS

HOW CAN I BE SURE I AM EATING A NUTRITIOUS DIET?

Consult the **FOOD FOUNDATION FOR FITNESS PYRAMID** below. Although it is not foolproof, you will be assured of meeting most of your nutrient requirements. We recommend eating at least the minimum number of servings of fruits and vegetables and whole grain breads and cereals, especially if you are to achieve a nutritious diet. Our Pyramid is based on the USDA's *The Food Guide Pyramid: A Guide to Daily Food Choices*.

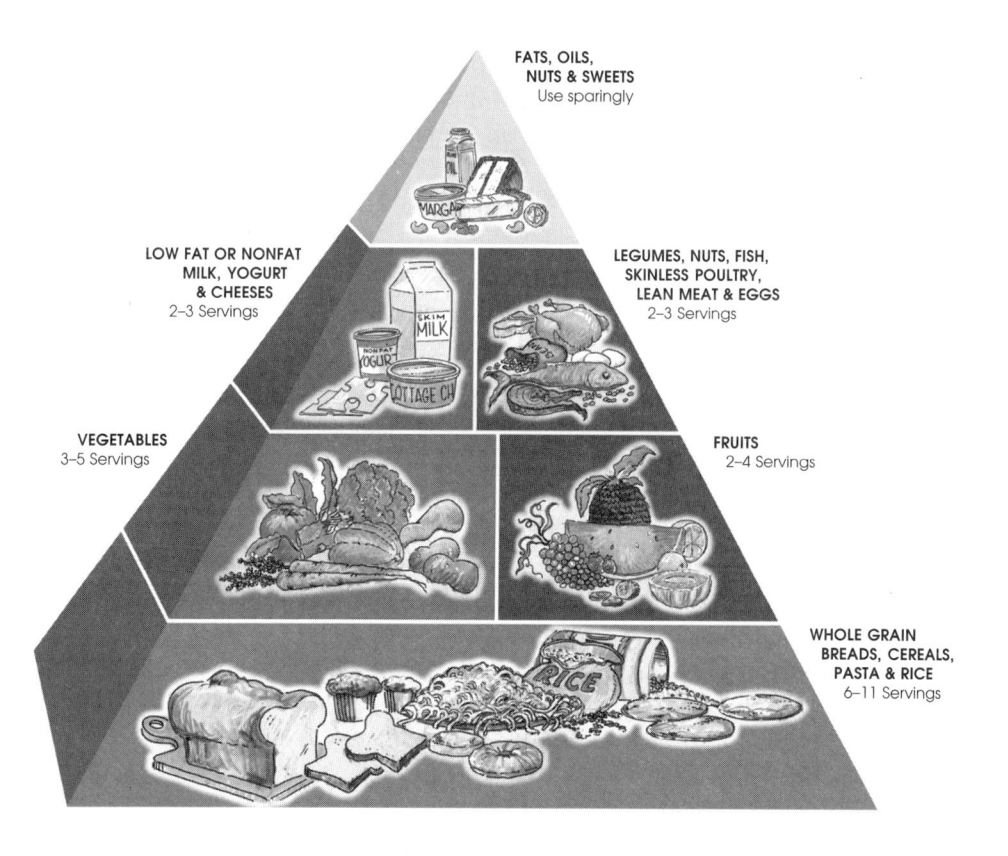

FOOD FOUNDATION FOR FITNESS PYRAMID

FATS, OILS, NUTS & SWEETS
Use sparingly

LOW FAT OR NONFAT MILK, YOGURT & CHEESES
2-3 Servings

LEGUMES, NUTS, FISH, SKINLESS POULTRY, LEAN MEAT & EGGS
2-3 Servings

VEGETABLES
3-5 Servings

FRUITS
2-4 Servings

WHOLE GRAIN BREADS, CEREALS, PASTA & RICE
6-11 Servings

Some of you will find the following chart helpful in determining how many servings of each food group to eat for different calorie levels.

NUMBER OF SERVINGS FOR VARIOUS CALORIE LEVELS

Food Group	Many Women Older Adults About 1600	Teenage Girls Active Women Most Men About 2200	Teenage Boys Active Men About 2800
Bread	6	9	11
Vegetable	3	4	5
Fruit	2	3	4
Milk**	2–3	2–3	2–3
Meat	2 (2.5 oz.)	2 (3 oz.)	2 (3.5 oz.)

**Women who are pregnant or breast feeding, teenagers, and young adults to age 24 need 3 servings.*

If you choose low fat, lean foods from the major food groups and use fat, oils and sweets sparingly, you can eat the number of servings from each food group shown above and not worry about counting fat grams.

MORE FOOD FOUNDATION FOR FITNESS GUIDELINES

1. Consume at least 50–60 percent of your calories from carbohydrates—grains, vegetables, fruits, low fat or skim milk products.

2. Increase fiber in your diet—more whole grain products, vegetables, fruits.

3. Eat less fat, saturated fat and cholesterol. This means eating more legumes, fish and poultry and choosing the leaner cuts of meat such as beef or pork. Reduce fat calories to 30 percent or less of total daily calorie intake.

4. Consume more fresh and minimally processed foods.

5. If you eat sugar-containing foods or alcohol, do so in moderation.

6. Eat at least three times a day. It is wise to avoid skipping meals. Recent evidence indicates snacking may be a positive habit.

7. Consume 1/2 to 2/3 of your day's intake before the evening meal.

8. Eat a variety of foods.

MORE ABOUT FIBER

Fiber is believed to be essential for good bowel health. Many authorities believe it may help prevent cancer of the bowel, as well as other problems such as hemorrhoids and diverticulosis. Remember, foods which are good sources of fiber are fruits, vegetables, legumes and whole grain cereal products. They are award winners since they contain little or no fat, lots of good nutrition and NO cholesterol.

The Pyramid recommendations on page 35 will help you obtain the desirable amount of fiber needed for good health. Face it, most of us do not eat enough fiber! To summarize these recommendations, you need 6–11 servings of whole grain bread and cereal products, 5–9 servings of fruits and vegetables, including legumes. OOPS, sorry, but juices usually don't count as fiber sources. Some of the popular juicing machines remove much of the fiber during the juicing process.

Inexperienced fiber eaters may want to ease into consuming all of the above recommended foods. Proceed cautiously! Fiber is famous for flatulence (intestinal gas)! You will feel better if you add one or two new foods at a time, rather than too much, too soon.

WARNING! You need plenty of water to prevent constipation on a higher fiber diet—at least 6 to 8 glasses of liquids daily.

MENU GUIDE

The following menu guide will show you what high carbohydrate, low fat meals look like. The fat level is below 30 percent of the calories and the carbohydrate level is above 50 percent of the calories. People who eat like this will be more nutritionally fit and will probably have less chance of developing heart disease and other chronic diseases. Please use this outline only as a means of making more informed selections of foods and don't view it as another "diet" you have to follow.

SPECIAL NOTE FOR USING MENU GUIDE:

We have suggested on the menu guide eating certain foods such as 2 slices of whole wheat bread. However, there may be times when you don't want bread. When this happens, select other carbohydrate-containing foods such as other cereal products or fruits or vegetables.

We did not list the fat grams for these meals because individual food choices will have some bearing on the fat gram total. Most of the time the fat content will be less than 30 percent of the calories. Notice how much food can be planned into 1600 calories. Keep in mind your needs may be different.

MENU GUIDE FOR APPROXIMATELY 1600 CALORIES
BREAKFAST
*1 egg, prepared without fat or 1 ounce low fat or part skim milk cheese
2 slices whole wheat toast (omit egg, if desired, and add 1 additional slice toast)
1 cup skim milk
12 ounces of citrus fruit juice or vegetable juice or 2 pieces of fresh fruit
1 teaspoon of margarine or 2 teaspoons of "diet" margarine

LUNCH
3 ounces very lean meat, fish or poultry, prepared without fat
1/2-1 cup green or yellow vegetables, prepared without fat
2 slices of whole wheat bread
1 piece of fresh fruit
2 teaspoons of margarine or mayonnaise or 4 teaspoons of "diet' margarine (for spread or cooking)

SNACK
1 cup dry cereal or 3/4 cup cooked cereal or 1 1/2 slices bread
1 cup skim milk
1 piece of fresh fruit

DINNER
3 ounces very lean meat, fish or poultry, prepared without fat
1 large baked potato or 1 cup corn, beans, pasta product or rice
1/2–1 cup green or yellow vegetables, prepared without fat
2 teaspoons regular margarine or 4 teaspoons "diet" margarine (for spread or cooking)

*To reduce cholesterol in the diet, you may want to limit egg yolks to no more than 3–4 per week.

NUTRITION QUALITY CHECK
Check out your food fitness, using the Pyramid guidelines. The food frequency diary on the next page will give you an idea about whether you are consuming a high quality diet. Make a tally mark under each food grouping when you have eaten a serving of food listed there. Continue for each meal and snack for a week. Total your tally marks for the entire week under the column labeled Weekly Totals. Mixed dishes such as chili or spaghetti will be marked under more than one grouping of food.

For example, if you eat the following dinner: 1 1/2 cups tuna noodle casserole (with skim milk white sauce) and 1 cup broccoli seasoned with 1 teaspoon of margarine, your tally sheet would look something like this:

1/2 Cup Cooked Rice, Pasta, Cereal	I I
1/2 Cup Chopped Raw Or Cooked Vegetable	I I
1 Cup Skim Milk Or Yogurt	1/2
2 Ounces Cooked Fish, Poultry, Lean Meat	I

NUTRITION QUALITY CHECK

TYPE OF FOOD	NUMBER OF SERVINGS	WEEKLY TOTALS	WEEKLY GOALS
GRAIN GROUP			42+
1 Slice Whole Grain Bread			
1/2 Bagel Or 1/2 English Muffin			
1 Tortilla Or 1 Pancake			
1/2 Cup Cooked Rice, Pasta, Cereal			
1 Ounce Ready-to-eat Cereal			
VEGETABLES			14–21
1/2 Chopped Raw Or Cooked Vegetables			
1 Cup Raw Leafy Vegetables			
FRUITS			35+
1 Piece Fruit Or Melon Wedge			
3/4 Cup Juice			
1/2 Cup Canned Fruit			
1/4 Cup Dried Fruit			
MILK, YOGURT AND CHEESE			14
1 Cup Of Lowfat Or Skim Milk Or Yogurt			
1 1/2 To 2 Ounces Of Cheese			
PROTEIN FOODS			14–21
2 Ounces Cooked Poultry, Fish Or Lean Meat			
Count 1/2 Cup Cooked Dried Beans, 1 Egg, 2 Tablespoons Of Peanut Butter Or 1/3 Cup Nuts As 1 Ounce Of Lean Meat			

Chapter 9

READY, SET, GO!!

The road to healthy eating habits is paved with good intentions which often go the way of New Year's resolutions. This usually happens because you probably attempted to do too much too soon. Typically, the person vowing to eat more healthily fails because the first day the diet changes is completely different from the way he/she was eating before. Let us help you with this hurdle—diet evolution instead of diet revolution. In other words, take a step at a time.

To illustrate, Gayle decided she wanted to reduce her body fat and learn to eat in a healthy way. Her past track record was not successful—losing and gaining weight with every diet. She knew there must be a better way.

When she came to see us, we suggested she record a few days of her normal food intake. This record would show her where she might need to improve her diet. What she found out was that she was eating an average of 1 serving per day of fruits/vegetables and and average of 3 servings per day of breads/cereals. Remember the Food Guide Pyramid goals are a minimum 5 servings of fruits/vegetables and a minimum 6 servings of bread/cereals. Gayle was horrified that she needed to eat 4 more servings of fruits/vegetables and 3 more bread/cereal servings each day.

We told her "not to worry". New habits need to be phased in a little at a time. To increase fruits and vegetables, she decided to eat 1 piece of fresh fruit each day for a mid-morning snack and to increase breads/cereals by eating 1/2 bagel in the afternoon when she was always hungry. Notice she did not try to change everything at once. These additions were her only goals the first week. After three weeks when this habit felt comfortable, she decided to add a bowl of cereal for breakfast and a vegetable serving at lunch. She practiced these habits until they took hold.

WHY CAN'T I JUST ADD ALL THE FOODS I NEED AT ONE TIME? IT WILL TAKE TOO LONG TO IMPROVE MY DIET IF I FOLLOW GAYLE'S EXAMPLE.
You could do this, but we predict you won't stay with the new habits very long. Give yourself a chance to gradually adapt each change to your diet—just as you gave your body a chance to adapt gradually to the exercise habit.

Eventually, Gayle met the goal of at least 5 servings of fruits/vegetables and 6 servings of breads/cereals a day. In the process of adding these healthy foods to her diet, she decreased some of the high fat foods she had been eating. A typical dinner for Gayle had been a large piece of meat and a salad with a lot of salad dressing. She added, over time, a serving of potato and a cooked vegetable. Then, she looked at the Pyramid and noticed that meat servings were about 2-3 ounces and she was eating 6-8 ounces for dinner. At that point, she decided she could save money and eat a smaller serving more in line with the Pyramid recommendations. She also decided to try a lower fat salad dressing and liked it. In the process, she cut the fat in her dinner meal by about 20–30 grams, a saving of 180–210 calories. All this without going on a "diet"!

We recommend you take a look at your intake and decide what additions, alterations and/or substitutions you need to make. Then decide the easiest small goal you can shoot for first and go for it.

ALL OF THIS SOUNDS GOOD, BUT I DON'T HAVE TIME TO COOK BREAKFAST OR FIX LUNCH NOW.

Good point! More people than ever are skipping meals because of time constraints. Let's look at how you can get out of this rut. Gayle was skipping both breakfast and lunch and eating non-stop after she got home from work. When this occurs, it is almost impossible to eat all the foods recommended for good health.

Here's how she worked on the problem. Gayle felt she could not handle eating breakfast and lunch immediately but believed she could handle snacks. She planned to purchase fruit and bagels on the weekend for her mid morning and mid afternoon snacks. **Planning** was the key. Know what you are going to eat and when.

One of the bigger nutrition myths is that we must sit down for three square meals a day. Not so! Many people who don't have time to eat a whole meal are finding "grazing" (eating many small snacks or meals) to be a healthy alternative and planning makes it possible.

WHO'S GOT THE TIME TO PLAN?

Gayle got very creative about making plans. She kept a grocery list going on her desk. If she found herself listening to music on phone hold, she jotted down a few items she needed. She also made food plans while she was going to and from work, while riding her exercise bicycle, while under the hair dryer and while watching TV. Use your imagination to come up with your own food planning times.

Adding an early morning snack in order to include all the healthy foods she needed became Gayle's next challenge in the evolution of her eating habits. She made a list of foods she would consider eating:

- Yogurt mixed with cereal and fruit
- Toast or bread, milk or yogurt, juice or fruit
- English muffin, jelly
- Leftovers from dinner
- Cottage cheese, crackers or toast
- Lowfat muffins, jelly
- Freezer waffles or pancakes
- Cereal, milk, juice or fruit
- Bagel, fat free cream cheese, fruit

Some people would choose a different item from their list every day. Gayle chose the easy route and decided an English muffin with jelly would be a good "starter" for her day. To save time and effort, she bought a half dozen packages of English muffins and froze them, along with another half dozen packages of bagels for her afternoon snack. Many people keep several types of bread products in the freezer.

She made another list of snack possibilities for quick grazing that could be stored at her desk or in her purse:
- Any type of bread—bagels, muffins, bread sticks, pita bread, rice cakes
- Fresh fruit
- Dried prunes, apricots, peaches, raisins, figs
- Juice—6 ounce cans or paper cartons
- Lowfat popcorn
- Lowfat crackers, lowfat cheese
- Raw vegetables
- Unsweetened cereal
- Mini cans of tuna, water packed
- Fig bars

WHAT CAN I DO IF I DECIDE TO EAT LUNCH?

Back to basics—planning. Here are some ideas Gayle tried when she decided to incorporate lunch into her schedule. She tried the basic brown bag first, then microwave meals, combinations of her stored snacks, cooking extra for dinner and bringing the leftovers for lunch, going out to fast food restaurants and selecting healthier choices using the food tables in the back of this book.

Gayle came to prefer the brown bag. Here's what she added to her grocery list. Remember she has an assortment of breads in the freezer.
- Low fat deli meats or packaged luncheon meats
- Mustard
- Fat free salad dressing (mayonnaise type)
- Fresh fruit—oranges, bananas, apples, cut up melons
- Raw vegetables from grocery salad bar
- Cottage cheese
- Yogurt

Gayle added a potato and vegetable to her evening meal, but needed more ideas for quick fixes for dinner. You might find the following ideas helpful, also. Stock your cupboards with staples such as pasta—several types, rice, canned vegetables, canned beans, canned soups (get lower sodium if salt is a concern), canned fruits. If you have a large enough freezer, add frozen vegetables, frozen dinners, frozen entrees—see the Food Value Table in the back of the book for fat, calorie and sodium content.

I'VE ALWAYS HEARD THAT CANNED FOODS ARE NOT GOOD FOR YOU.

Canned foods retain as much of their nutritional value as cooked fresh ones. Maybe more. Frozen and canned foods are processed at their peak and have not been hanging around the grocery or your refrigerator for a week or so, losing some of their vitamin content.

HOW ABOUT A GROCERY LIST THAT I COULD JUST FILL OUT EACH WEEK?

All you had to do was ask. Feel free to make copies and take them with you when you shop.

GROCERY LIST

Breads (Bagel, Pita, Raisin, White, Wh Wh)
_____
_____

Buns
_____

Tortilla/Taco Shells
Crackers, Lowfat
_____

Cereal, Cold/Hot
_____
_____

Crackers, Lowfat
_____
_____

Muffins-English/Lowfat
_____

Pasta-Macaroni/Spaghetti
_____

Pasta-Boxed Mixes
_____

Rice-Brown/White
_____

Rice-Boxed Mixes
_____

Frozen Pancakes/Waffles
_____
_____

Beans, Canned/Dry
_____
_____
_____

Vegetables, Fresh
_____
_____

Fruit, Fresh
_____
_____

Vegetables/Fruits, Canned
_____
_____
_____

Juice-Vegetable/Fruit, Canned/Frozen
_____
_____

Lean Beef/Pork
_____
_____

Chicken/Turkey
_____
_____

Fish, Fresh/Frozen
_____
_____

Canned Fish/Poultry/Meat
_____

Peanut Butter, Lowfat
_____

Cheese, Lowfat
_____
_____

Staples-Flour/Sugar/Oil/
Fat Free Salad Dressing
_____
_____
_____

Milk, Lowfat/Skim
_____

Yogurt, Lowfat
_____

Frozen Dinners/Items
_____
_____
_____

Condiments/Spices/Herbs
_____
_____

Other Beverages
_____
_____

Miscellaneous
_____
_____
_____
_____
_____
_____
_____
_____
_____

Margarine/Other Spreads
_____
_____

Chapter 10

FIRST YOU SAY WE CAN AND THEN WE CAN'T
(Sorting Out the Conflicting Information About Controlling Blood Cholesterol)

I NEED TO WATCH MY CHOLESTEROL AND SATURATED FAT INTAKE, BUT DON'T REALLY KNOW WHAT THESE TERMS MEAN.

No problem. Just remember that cholesterol is a waxy, fat-like substance found **only** in animal foods. It is essential for many body functions. Even if you didn't eat any cholesterol, your liver would make enough for your body's needs. Saturated fat, on the other hand, is found in foods of both animal and plant origins. Usually, saturated fat is solid at room temperature.

WHY DO I NEED TO BE CONCERNED ABOUT CHOLESTEROL AND SATURATED FAT INTAKE?

A high blood level of cholesterol is a major contributor to developing hardening of the arteries (collections of hardened fat, cholesterol and debris on the inner walls of the arteries.) This condition, called atherosclerosis, can lead to heart attacks or strokes. High levels of cholesterol and saturated fat in the diet do tend to increase blood levels of cholesterol in **some** people. However, a high **saturated fat** intake is the biggest culprit in causing cholesterol levels to increase.

I AM SO CONFUSED ABOUT WHAT I CAN AND CAN'T EAT TO HELP LOWER THE CHOLESTEROL IN MY BLOOD.

We don't blame you for being confused. Many health professionals feel the same way. The flood of current research, instead of clearing up our confusion, only seems to add to it. Several years back we recommended that people increase the amount of polyunsaturated fatty acids (PUFAs) in their diets to lower their blood cholesterol. These PUFAs are found in oils such as safflower, sunflower and corn. People went around dutifully adding several teaspoons per day of these oils to their food.

The monounsaturated fatty acids (MUFAs) were thought to have no effect on cholesterol levels in the blood. MUFAs are found in canola, olive and peanut oils. The group of fatty acids that had a "bad" reputation were the saturated fatty acids (SFAs) found in animal foods and tropical oils such as palm, palm kernel and coconut. SFAs and dietary cholesterol itself were blamed for increasing the level of cholesterol in the blood. So, diets were restricted in cholesterol and the SFAs. Since the so-called "red" meats and dairy products contained high levels of SFAs and cholesterol, they were severely limited or banned. Tropical oils were also prohibited and shellfish were a "NO-NO" because of an apparent high cholesterol content.

Now, we are recommending the use of oils high in MUFAs for cooking because some research indicates MUFAs help lower total cholesterol in the blood without lowering the "good" cholesterol known as high density lipoproteins (HDLs). PUFAs lower total cholesterol but appear to lower the "good" HDLs, as well. Shellfish are back on the menu because chemical analyses have become more precise and the cholesterol content was not as high as first thought.

Currently controversy whirls around the tropical oils and **some** SFAs which may not be the "bad" guys they once were thought to be. Also, some authorities contend that dietary cholesterol may or may not affect blood cholesterol, depending on the individual's response to it.

IN THE MIDST OF ALL THIS CONFUSION, WHAT DO I DO?

We support the dietary guidelines from such prestigious health organizations as The American Heart Association (AHA), The American Cancer Society, The American Diabetes Association, and The American Dietetic Association to lower total fat in the diet to 20-30 percent of calories. The reasons these health organizations believe we need to be stingier with fat in our diets are that certain forms of heart disease and cancers are associated with a high fat intake. We also know most people with diabetes can have better health if they decrease their fat intake, especially SFAs.

Reducing fat in the diet will automatically reduce your intake of all PUFAs, MUFAs and SFAs. We also believe that until the research dust settles, limiting intake of foods high in SFAs is a good idea. See TABLE 10-4 on page 50 for the PUFA, MUFA and SFA content of the various types of fat. As for the cholesterol level in the diet, we suggest staying with AHA's recommendation of 300 or fewer milligrams of dietary cholesterol per day.

We believe you can achieve your health goals by lowering your intake of total fat (with or without calorie counting), minimizing sugar and alcohol intake and eating a diet high in vegetables, fruits, cereal grains and legumes.

WHAT IS A GOOD LEVEL FOR MY CHOLESTEROL?

Excellent question—everyone should know what their cholesterol reading is, including young people. The following table will help you know where you stand.

	TOTAL CHOLESTEROL LEVELS	
DESIRABLE	**BORDERLINE–HIGH**	**TOO HIGH**
Less than 200 mg/dl	200–239 mg/dl	Over 239 mg/dl

Even more important than total cholesterol level is the ratio of your HDLs to that total. For example, Max had a total cholesterol level of 250 mg/dl, but his HDL level was 80 mg/dl for a ratio of 3.1. (divide the total cholesterol by the amount of the HDL). A desirable ratio is 4.5 or below. The best ratios are 3.5 or below. His doctors patted him on the back and told him he was in good shape. The point is, it is **not** enough to know only the total cholesterol figure. You need to find out your HDL and your LDL levels too.

The **higher** your level of HDL cholesterol, "the right stuff", the **lower** your risk of heart disease. The **higher** your LDL level, "the wrong stuff", the **greater** your risk of heart disease.

LDL CHOLESTEROL LEVELS		
DESIRABLE	**BORDERLINE–HIGH**	**TOO HIGH**
Less than 130 mg/dl	130–159 mg/dl	160 mg/dl or more

LDL levels are lowered by decreasing cholesterol and saturated fat intake in the diet. HDL levels are increased by exercising, quitting smoking, and decreasing body fat.

When you eat a diet low in total fat, your cholesterol and saturated fat intake are decreased automatically. It is usually enough just to count total fat grams in your diet and follow the guidelines presented in this chapter.

I WOULD LIKE TO KNOW WHAT IT ACTUALLY MEANS TO HAVE A 20 TO 30 PERCENT FAT INTAKE.

We know some of you who started at the beginning of the book already know what is meant by a 20–30 percent intake of fat. For those of you who are just interested in lowering your blood cholesterol and may have started the book with this chapter, we will repeat. Here goes!

Because most people do not go around with a dietitian in their hip pocket, this guideline to lower fat to 20 or 30 percent of calories can be a confusing one; most dietitians would prefer not to be bothered with all of these mathematical computations, either, if the truth were known.

Look no further! Help is at hand! You do not need to be a math whiz to be able to eat the recommended level of fat in your diet.

If you want to be more precise and figure your fat grams based on 20–30 percent of your calorie needs, as most dietary guidelines suggest, then you will need to know your estimated daily calorie needs.

HOW MANY CALORIES DO I NEED?

You won't know exactly because your calorie needs are influenced by your physical activity level and inherited factors.

We have chosen to base our calorie guidelines on information presented in the 1989 edition of *RECOMMENDED DIETARY ALLOWANCES*. These guidelines are based on people engaging in very light, sedentary activities. Your own calorie needs may vary, but, for purposes of figuring your desired fat intake, these guidelines are close enough.
So, here's a table to help you in computing daily calorie needs to arrive at your daily fat intake.

TABLE 10-1
CALORIES PER POUND BASED ON AGE

Ages 15–18	16
Ages 19–24	14
Ages 25–50	13
Ages 51+	12

For example, Connie, who is 40 and weighs 150 pounds, has an estimated calorie need of about 1950 per day. We calculated her calories this way: 13 x 150 = 1950. Or, Max, who is 55 and weighs 175 pounds, needs approximately 2100 calories (12 x 175 = 2100).

You will need to find the number of calories per pound opposite your age on the table above and multiply this number times your weight in pounds.

DOES THIS MEAN I HAVE TO COUNT CALORIES, TOO?

No! You only did this calculation so you could figure your desirable number of fat grams per day. It so happens we have concocted an easy to use "do-it-yourself" table. See below.

TABLE 10-2
DAILY LEVELS OF CALORIES AND FAT

Calories	Fat Grams (30% of Calories)	(20% of Calories)
1400	46	31
1500	50	33
1600	54	36
1700	56	38
1800	60	40
1900	64	42
2000	66	44
2100	70	47
2200	74	49
2300	78	51
2400	80	53
2500	84	56
2600	87	58
2700	90	60
2800	93	62
2900	97	64
3000	100	67

For example, Connie set 65 grams of fat as her daily intake if she aims for a fat intake of 30% of her estimated need of 1950 calories. If she lowers her fat intake to 20 percent of her calories, she can eat about 43 grams of fat. Our advice is for Connie (or you) to begin at the 30 percent level and, if necessary, gradually reduce your fat intake to the 20 percent level.

A good rule of thumb is to aim for 35–50 or fewer fat grams per day if you are a gal and 40–60 if you are a guy. You will most likely be consuming a lower fat and healthier diet than you are now.

GUIDELINES TO LOWERING CHOLESTEROL IN THE DIET

When you look at the food tables, be aware that any food which is animal in origin, alone or in combination with other foods, will have some cholesterol content. The potato which has been seasoned with cheese or butter is a good example. If the food is low in total fat content, it is probably no problem for you even if it contains some cholesterol. Exceptions include egg yolks and organ meats, which are moderate in fat content but contain much more cholesterol than even "red" meat.

The American Heart Association has recommended keeping cholesterol intake below 300 milligrams per day. To accomplish this goal, use skim milk (even 1–2 percent milk has fat and cholesterol) and other low or no fat dairy products. Limit egg yolk intake to four per week and organ meat intake to one or fewer times per month. Keep intake of **lean** meat, fish or skinless poultry to four to six ounces per day.

To see if your cholesterol intake falls within these guidelines, use the chart below.

TABLE 10-3
CHOLESTEROL COMPARISON CHECK

FOOD	MILLIGRAMS OF CHOLESTEROL
Fruits, Vegetables, Grains	0
Nuts, Seeds	0
Vegetable Oils	0
Egg Whites	0
Skim Milk/Skim Milk Yogurt (1 cup)	4
Buttermilk (1 cup)	9
Whole Milk (1 cup)	35
1% Fat Cottage Cheese (1 cup)	10
Creamed Cottage Cheese (1 cup)	31
Oysters, Cooked (About 3.5 oz.)	45
Fish, Lean Or Clams, Cooked (About 3.5 oz.)	65
Chicken/Turkey, Light Meat, Cooked, Without Skin (About 3.5 oz.)	80
Chicken/Turkey, Dark Meat, Cooked, Without Skin (About 3.5 oz.)	95
Beef, Lean, Cooked (About 3.5 oz.)	84

CHOLESTEROL COMPARISON CHECK

FOOD	MILLIGRAMS OF CHOLESTEROL
Lobster, Cooked (About 3.5 oz.)	85
Crab, Cooked (About 3.5 oz.)	100
Pork, Lean, Cooked (About 3.5 oz.)	111
Mozzarella, Part Skim (1 oz.)	17
Shrimp, Cooked (About 3.5 oz.)	150
Cheddar Cheese (1 oz.)	30
Cream Cheese (1 oz.)	31
Egg Yolk (1 yolk)	211
Heavy Whipping Cream (1/4 cup)	82
Beef Liver, Cooked (About 3.5 oz.)	389
Chicken Livers, Cooked (About 3.5 oz.)	631
Beef Kidney, Cooked (About 3.5 oz.)	700
Butter (1 oz.)	62

GUIDELINES TO LOWER SATURATED FAT IN THE DIET

In general, choose polyunsaturated or monounsaturated oils or fats which are liquid at room temperature. On the label, look for the word hydrogenated, which means that a polyunsaturated vegetable fat has been turned into a partially saturated fat by adding hydrogen. In addition, until further research is in, beware of three liquid vegetable fats: coconut, palm and palm kernel oil. These are naturally highly saturated fats and are frequently used in the preparation of many convenience and fast foods. Cereals, crackers, microwave popcorn, and many frozen ready-to-heat products are some of the most notorious sources of these oils. READ LABELS!!! See Chapter 13 on page 58 for further label reading guidance.

When you do decide to use fat, some choices are better than others. Mono and polyunsaturated fats such as olive, canola, safflower or sunflower oil, along with corn oil, are the best choices. Other good oils are cottonseed, sesame seed and soybean. Use a light hand when adding any fat to your cooking or you may find you have exceeded your fat gram goal. See the OILS AND FATS chart on the next page for comparing types of fats.

TABLE 10-4
OILS AND FATS—KNOW THE DIFFERENCES!!!

The fatty acid values are given as percentages of total fat and may not add up to 100 percent due to the presence of other fat substances in the oil.

Type of Fat or Oil	Polyunsaturated	Monounsaturated	Saturated
Safflower Oil	74%	12%	9%
Sunflower Oil	65%	20%	10%
Corn Oil	59%	24%	13%
Soybean Oil	58%	24%	14%
Cottonseed Oil	52%	18%	26%
Canola Oil	30%	59%	7%
Olive Oil	8%	73%	13%
Peanut Oil	32%	46%	17%
Soft Tub Margarine, Typical	61%	18%	16%
Stick Margarine, Typical	32%	45%	18%
Vegetable Shortening	14%	51%	30%
Palm Oil	10%	37%	49%
Coconut Oil	2%	6%	87%
Palm Kernel Oil	2%	11%	82%
Cocoa Butter	3%	33%	60%
Tuna Fat	63%	?-	27%
Turkey Fat	23%	43%	30%
Chicken Fat	21%	45%	30%
Goose Fat	11%	57%	27%
Duck Fat	13%	49%	34%
Lard	11%	45%	39%
Mutton Fat	8%	41%	48%
Beef Fat	4%	41%	50%
Butter Fat	5%	30%	62%

 Notice that the fats with the highest percentages of saturated fatty acids, the "bad" stuff, are listed toward the bottom of the chart. The worst animal fat offenders appear to be mutton, beef, and butter fat (found in full fat dairy products). Don't get dairy products containing butter fat confused with low fat or fat free dairy products such as skim milk and fat free cheese and yogurt. These low fat dairy foods are necessary for a healthy diet.
 To complicate the controversies surrounding MUFAs, PUFAs, and SFAs, there are also fatty acids known as "cis" and "trans". Margarines contain "trans" fatty acids due to the partial hydrogenation (saturation) process they undergo to keep them from being liquid. "Trans" fatty acids elevate blood LDL cholesterol. So what is a person to do, go back to butter? Until more facts are in, most experts believe margarine is still a better choice than

butter, especially if you choose one that has a liquid oil (one that is low in SFA) listed as the first ingredient. The moral to this story is continue to follow a diet low in all types of fat.

I KEEP HEARING THAT OMEGA-3 OR EPA CAPSULES ARE A GOOD THING TO TAKE TO LOWER MY CHOLESTEROL.

Research shows that Eskimos who have a high intake of Omega-3 fatty acids (found in fish oils) have low cholesterol levels and a low incidence of heart disease. The effectiveness of EPA capsules in lowering cholesterol is not proven, and some authorities have found problems with their use. You certainly need to contact your physician before taking these capsules. Most experts believe that the best way for you to increase your intake of these important fatty acids is to eat two or more fish meals per week.

WHAT IF MY TRIGLYCERIDES ARE HIGH TOO?

Triglycerides come from the fats in our foods and if blood levels are too high (above 200 mg/dl), you may be at risk for developing heart disease. Losing body fat, lowering dietary fat, and eating more fruits, vegetables, whole grains and legumes are the best things you can do to lower triglyceride levels—in other words, following the same guidelines that are recommended for lowering cholesterol.

Usually, reducing intake of high sugar foods and alcoholic beverages also helps. Discuss your individual health concerns with your dietitian or physician.

LIFE AFTER FAT COOKING TIPS

Invest in the nonstick varieties of skillets. Yes, they really do fry chicken without fat. Use non stick pan sprays to help keep food from sticking in any pan or skillet.

If you must use oil or fat, you'd be surprised how little you need. If a recipe calls for 2 tablespoons of fat, 1 teaspoon is enough to sauté your onions, garlic or whatever. Use vermouth or other dry white wine, burgundy, broth, tomato or vegetable juice cocktail for "sautéing" vegetables or meats. Add herbs and spices to your heart's content. "French fried" oven fried potato sticks are easier to prepare than regular deep-fat fried ones. One teaspoon of oil sprinkled over 2 sliced potatoes on a cookie sheet will produce tasty "fries". Sprinkle with paprika and onion powder.

Try out this recipe. "Sauté" any vegetable or mix of vegetables such as zucchini squash, cherry tomatoes, onions, mushrooms, green peppers, broccoli, or carrot strips in 1/2 cup vermouth or burgundy, 1/4 teaspoon each of garlic powder and onion powder, and 1/2 teaspoon bouillon granules until the liquid is cooked down. Salt (if not restricted) and pepper to taste. Variation: Add soy sauce, lemon juice or Worcestershire Sauce in place of the bouillon.

PREPARING MEAT, POULTRY, FISH

Buy leaner cuts of meat such as rump roast or round steak or pork loin. Trim off all visible fat from any cut before cooking. Skin all poultry BEFORE eating. Buy water-packed tuna instead of oil packed. You'll save fat grams.

Panbroil without fat. Use wine for cooking, if desired, unless you have a problem with alcohol. Cooking does evaporate some, but not all the alcohol, depending on the method of cooking.

Broiling in the oven or outdoors helps get rid of more fat. Marinades for barbecuing, broiling or baking, which use lemon juice, wine, whiskey, vinegar, spices, and herbs tenderize and add flavor. Omit the oil or fat called for—you'll never miss it.

SAUCES, GRAVIES

Gravy can be made with any defatted meat broth and 2 tablespoons flour or corn starch dissolved in cold water and mixed with the simmering broth to make 1 cup. Before making gravy, always let meat broth sit in the refrigerator until the fat comes to the top. Skim it off. Use the same technique for sauces.

Can't throw out those leftovers? Try the best soup ever. This is one way to get rid of a habit many people have—cleaning up all the leftovers after a meal by eating them. So if you can't bring yourself to "waste" them instead of "waisting" them, try this. For those dibs and dabs of this and that which have been so tempting to eat instead of throwing out, start a soup pot in your freezer. Add that spoon of green beans, potatoes, any other vegetable, leftover meat broth, defatted meat scraps, rice, etc. which you can't bring yourself to part with. When you have enough scraps in your freezer for a meal, thaw, add broth or tomato juice, if necessary, and you will have some of the tastiest soup ever.

Chapter 11

SALT, SALT EVERYWHERE AND NOTHING LEFT TO EAT

- Are you perplexed about what's left to eat when you've been told you can't have salt?

- Are you confused about the difference between salt and sodium?

- Are you fed up with foods that taste blah after you've shaken the salt habit?

- If you answered "yes" to any of the above questions, this section is for you.

SALT IS IN EVERYTHING!
This is doubtless your impression if you've read many labels in the grocery store recently. See Chapter 13 on page 58 for more information on label reading. Salt is the second most popular food additive in this country; sugar is first. Salt is composed of two minerals, sodium and chloride. Sodium, approximately 40 percent of salt, is the real culprit if you're trying to reduce salt in your diet. The sodium in foods is usually measured in milligrams. A milligram is 1/1000 of a gram. To put this into perspective, a gram is about the weight of a paper clip. Low sodium diets prescribed by physicians ordinarily are 2–3 grams of sodium a day. This means total food eaten during a day's time should contain no more than 2000 or 3000 milligrams of sodium.

One way of staying within the prescribed limit is to consult the **TABLE OF FOOD VALUES** beginning on page 64 which shows the sodium content of foods and then to add up milligrams of sodium in each kind and amount of food eaten. Another way to limit your sodium intake is to use a prepared list of "dos and dont's". We believe such a list is too restrictive and does not allow you to make informed choices of the foods you eat.

HERE'S HOW YOU "CAN HAVE" SOME OF THOSE FOODS YOU NEVER THOUGHT YOU'D EAT AGAIN AND STILL CONTROL SODIUM INTAKE.
We can't promise you a pickle binge, but you'll be surprised at what you "can have" and still be within safe sodium limits. You may have to ignore the lists of "forbidden" foods provided by most low sodium diets and be willing to engage in some creative choosing and a little arithmetic.

The ham you've longed for might still be yours! Salt cured ham is generally considered one of the most menacing foods in a low sodium diet. But, consider this: 1 ounce of lean ham is worth 340 milligrams of sodium. Should you decide to eat 1 ounce of ham with your navy beans, this still leaves a reasonably generous 1660 sodium milligrams for the rest of the day if your prescribed level of sodium is 2000 milligrams. Even salt can be used with caution. A carefully measured level one-fourth teaspoon of salt will cost you about 575 sodium milligrams. If you choose to work salt into your prescribed sodium milligrams, we would recommend putting the day's measured amount in your own private salt shaker. If you have some left over, it should **not** be added to the next day's ration. Discard any leftover salt and start fresh the next day.

READ ALL LABELS.

Salt is not the only place where sodium is found. A brief glance at any grocery shelf will reveal an abundance of other compounds containing sodium. It is wise to avoid eating any food which has any of the following ingredients added **unless** you know the number of sodium milligrams for that particular food: salt, baking soda, baking powder, disodium phosphate, sodium alginate, sodium benzoate, sodium hydroxide, sodium proprionate, sodium sulfite, and monosodium glutamate. With the newer food labels, knowing the sodium content is easier than ever.

NUTRIENT INSURANCE

Counting sodium milligrams is important but there are about 40 other nutrients that count too. You could choose to spend all of your sodium budget for pickles, olives and corned beef, but this might not leave you enough to spare for all of the foods essential for good health. To insure an adequate intake of these nutrients, consume all the foods recommended in Chapter 8 on page 35. You will find yourself eating more vegetables, fruits and whole grain or enriched breads and cereals which improve your odds of getting a nutritionally adequate diet. Fortunately, fresh or frozen fruits and vegetables without salt or sugar added are nutritional giants as well as low sodium bargains.

SPECIAL NOTE FOR PEOPLE WITH HYPERTENSION (HIGH BLOOD PRESSURE)

Your sodium intake is not the whole story! Many people who lose 5 or 10 pounds have been able to reduce their need for medication. Exercise can be a big boon here as well, aiding in body fat loss. For more information on this topic, read the chapters on exercise and decreasing fat in your diet in the first part of this book.

POTASSIUM

Some medicines that are prescribed for high blood pressure deplete the body of potassium, an essential mineral. For this reason, some of you may need to eat a diet rich in potassium. You should consult your physician, however, before increasing potassium in your diet since some types of kidney disease can cause too much potassium to build up in your system.

Some salt substitutes are high in potassium. You will want to consult your physician before using these to season your foods. Fruits, vegetables, fluid milks and yogurt are excellent potassium sources. Actually, some studies suggest that a diet high in potassium and low in sodium is protective against high blood pressure.

CALCIUM AND MAGNESIUM

Recently, some authorities have stressed the importance of adequate intakes of calcium and magnesium in all of our diets, particularly for those people with high blood pressure. These three minerals—potassium, calcium and magnesium—and their relationship to high blood pressure are areas of continuing research.

Foods high in calcium are dairy products (use low or nonfat dairy products) and green leafy vegetables. Foods high in magnesium are dried peas and beans, nuts, whole grain cereals, cocoa, chocolate and green leafy vegetables.

It turns out your mother was right, "drink your milk and eat your vegetables, fruits and whole grain breads and cereals."

SPECIAL NOTE:

The 1989 edition of the *RECOMMENDED DIETARY ALLOWANCES* has set 500 milligrams of sodium per day as the minimum requirement.

MAKE INFORMED CHOICES.

Just as with the fat and calorie information, we hope you will use the sodium information to make informed choices of foods. Use generous amounts of herbs, spices and lemon juice to season foods. One client made up a basket of condiments he could sprinkle on at the table when he needed to add zip to something he was eating. The basket included garlic and onion powder, seasoned pepper, tabasco sauce, a plastic squeeze bottle of lemon juice, an herb and spice blend, plus dill weed and a few other of his favorite herbs. Let your imagination be your guide!

Chapter 12

PLANNING A DIET FOR PEOPLE WITH DIABETES

The following guidelines are the backbone of healthy food choices for people with diabetes mellitus. They are the same guidelines we recommend for everybody. In other words, the foods you need for good health are the same foods your family needs for good health.

IF YOU ARE OVERFAT, READ THE CHAPTERS ON LOSING BODY FAT.
One of the best ways to decrease blood glucose (sugar) is to decrease body fat. Often, just a few pounds less of body fat can make a big difference. Exercise is the bottom line. So, if you have an elevated blood sugar level and are overfat, consult your physician and dietitian or other diabetes educator before proceeding with an exercise program. The first part of this book can provide a good starter guide for you. We have a list of recommended readings in Appendix B on page 139 which will give you more information about diabetes than is possible in this small book.

If you have a calorie prescription from your doctor or dietitian, use the fat and calorie information in Chapter 7 and in the food tables.

AVOID SKIPPING MEALS.
A minimum of three meals per day is recommended. You will probably find an afternoon and/or evening snack desirable. Discuss your best meal and snack distribution with a Registered Dietitian or other certified diabetes educator. Eat your meals and snacks at regular times every day. If you skip a meal or snack, you will probably find yourself overeating at the next eating opportunity.

Plan to eat about the same amount of food each day.

Learning to do home glucose monitoring will give you the needed information about when you need food and the effect certain foods or combinations of foods have on your blood sugar. In other words, you can be in control of your own food choices.

EAT MORE HIGH FIBER FOODS AND LESS SUGAR AND FAT!
The good news is . . . your diet is composed of ordinary foods. Research shows that a diet that is high in fiber and low in fat helps control blood sugar and lowers cholesterol and triglycerides in the blood. People with diabetes have an increased risk of heart disease, so lowering blood levels of both cholesterol and triglycerides is highly desirable. Consult Chapter 10 for guidelines on lowering cholesterol and triglycerides.

A DIET TO CONTROL BLOOD GLUCOSE IS:
  I. Varied in the kinds of foods eaten each day.
  See the recommendations on the **FOOD FOUNDATION FOR FITNESS PYRAMID** in Chapter 8 beginning on page 35.
  II. High in fiber. Increase fiber by:
   a. Eating fruits instead of juice whenever possible.
   b. Eating whole wheat or whole grain breads or cereals instead of white bread or refined cereals.
   c. Eating a minimum of 1–2 servings of vegetables or fruits at each lunch and dinner.
  III. Low in total fat. Several things can be done to accomplish this:
   a. Keep total fat grams below 35–50 per day if you are a woman or below 40–60 grams per day if you are a man. For more details on keeping fat intake at 20–30 percent of your calorie intake, read Chapters 7 and 10.
   b. Limit fish, poultry, and meat servings to 2–3 ounces at a meal.
   c. Consume more fish and skinned poultry, rather than "red" meat.
   d. Avoid high fat meats such as luncheon meats, bacon or sausage as often as possible.
   e. Eliminate fat in recipes or cut down on amounts given.
   f. Use lower fat salad dressings, lower calorie margarines, etc.
   g. Use skim milk instead of whole milk and lower fat cheeses instead of those with a higher fat content.
   h. Bake, broil and stew, rather than fry. "Sauté" in dry white or red wines, bouillon or tomato juice instead of oils or other fats.
   i. Use non stick pan sprays for frying.

REMEMBER, CONSULT CHAPTERS 7 AND 10 FOR MORE INFORMATION ON FAT, FIBER AND CALORIES. FOR INFORMATION ON SODIUM, CONSULT CHAPTER 11. THE FOOD VALUE TABLES CONTAIN INFORMATION ON ALL THREE.

Chapter 13

THE FOOD LABEL: WHAT'S ON IT AND HOW TO USE IT

In 1994, a new food label appeared on food packages. Consumers found it presented more useful, complete and accurate information than previous labels. See the sample label below. Does it look familiar? For those of you who already know how to use this label, you can skip this chapter. But, if you need some clarification, read on! To help you use the information on the label to the fullest, we will describe each section separately.

Nutrition Facts

Serving Size 1 cup (228 g)
Servings Per Container 2

Amount per Serving

Calories 250   Calories from Fat 110

	% Daily Value*
Total Fat 12g	**18%**
Saturated Fat 3g	**15%**
Cholesterol 30mg	**10%**
Sodium 470mg	**20%**
Total Carbohydrate 31g	**10%**
Dietary Fiber 0g	**0%**
Sugars 5g	
Protein 5g	

Vitamin A 4%	•	Vitamin C 2%
Calcium 20%	•	Iron 4%

*Percent Daily Values are based on a 2,000 calorie diet. Your daily values may be higher or lower depending on your calorie needs:

	Calories:	2,000	2,500
Total Fat	Less than	65g	80g
Sat Fat	Less than	20g	25g
Cholesterol	Less than	200mg	300mg
Total Carbohydrate		300g	375g
Dietary Fiber		25g	30g

Calories per gram:
Fat 9   •   Carbohydrate 4   •   Protein 4

Label Requirements — These dietary components are required for all food labels.

Nutrition Facts
The Food and Drug Administration (FDA) is responsible for all food labeling except meat and poultry.

Serving Size
This quantity is an important reference point since all calorie and nutrient information is based on the amount in one serving. Look for two measurements—common household—1 cup in our example and metric measures—228 g.

Servings Per Container
In this example, the package has **2** servings.

Amount per Serving
The amount of each nutrient listed in **one** serving.

Calories
This product has 250 calories in one serving—110 of these calories are from fat.

%Daily Value
%Daily Values (DV) show how much of the recommended amount of the nutrients listed are in one serving. These %DV are for a person needing 2,000 calories a day. %Daily Values are different if you need more or fewer calories.

A high %DV means the food contains a lot of a nutrient; a low %DV means it contains only a little.

You can use the %DV to compare foods. One product may show it provides 30% DV of fat. A "slimmed down" version of the same item might contain 10%DV of fat. You make the choice.

Vitamins and Minerals
Only the %DV for these four vitamins and minerals are required to be shown on a label. A manufacturer may voluntarily list others.

This product is a good source of calcium but would not be considered a good source of Vitamins A and C and Iron.

Uniform definitions for terms are used to describe products such as free, low, light (or lite), reduced, less, high, lean, extra lean, more and good sources of. You may be interested in these definitions. Here's what they mean.

LABEL CLAIM	DEFINITION—PER SERVING
Free	Product contains none or insignificant amounts of nutrient listed
Low	Low fat = 3 or less grams Low saturated fat=1 or less gram Low sodium=less than 140 milligrams Very low sodium=less than 35 milligrams Low cholesterol=less than 20 milligrams Low calorie=40 or less calories
Light (Lite)	Has 1/3 fewer calories or 1/2 the fat of the original 50% less sodium than the original
Reduced or Less	25% fewer calories or nutrients than the original
High	20% or more of the Daily Value (DV) for that nutrient
Lean	Per 100 grams: Less than 10 grams fat Less than 4 grams of saturated fat Less than 95 milligrams of cholesterol
Extra Lean	Per 100 grams: Less than 5 grams fat Less than 2 grams of saturated fat Less than 95 milligrams of cholesterol
More or Good Source Of	One of the nutrients is 10% or above the DV for the original

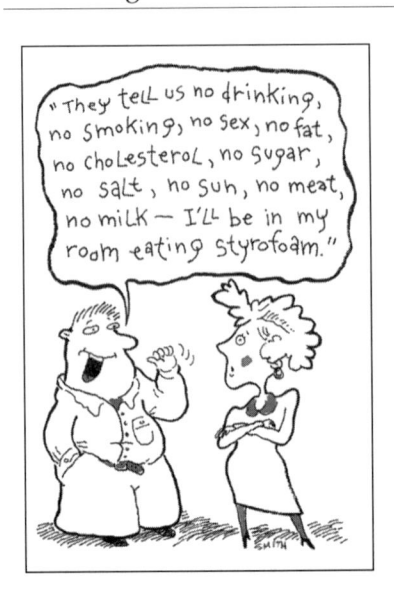

Chapter 14

HOW TO SUCCEED WHILE REALLY TRYING!

We thought it might be helpful to recap some tips about maintaining your new healthy habits—exercising and eating more fruits, vegetables, whole grain cereal products and less fat. We have dropped some hints along the way and felt that collecting them together along with a few new ones would help you in your quest for success.

1. **MODESTY BECOMES YOU!**

    Setting realistic, achievable goals is the first hallmark of success. The second is being able to evaluate your goals and set new ones if the old ones don't work. Turn mistakes into a learning experience rather than bashing yourself with the old failure "tapes".

2. **FIND OUT HOW FAT YOU ARE.**

    Knowing your body fat percentage is helpful in setting realistic eating and exercise goals.

3. **LISTEN TO AND GET TO KNOW YOUR BODY.**

    Eat when you are physically hungry and not for some of the other reasons people eat such as boredom, anger, depression, habit, time of day, etc. To eat when you are physically hungry, you need to recognize symptoms of physical hunger. These might be a growling stomach, headache, shakiness, tiredness, and sometimes anxiety (not situational).

    When it comes to exercise, do, but don't overdo. Know when to take a day off or when to stop your exercise session. If you feel very tired and don't know if you should go ahead and exercise, start slowly for 10 minutes. If you do not feel better after 10 minutes, give yourself permission to stop. If you do feel better, carry on!

4. **EAT AT LEAST THREE WELL-BALANCED MEALS A DAY.**

    Eating regularly and not skipping meals is a good way to avoid food cravings and possibly bingeing. High carbohydrate and fiber containing foods such as starchy foods, fruits and vegetables are particularly helpful.

    Some researchers have found that a carbohydrate snack in late afternoon serves most of us well and can help us avoid overeating at dinner and at night. Many of our clients who have followed this advice were able to stop overeating at night.

5. **PLEASE DON'T VIEW YOUR NEW EXERCISE AND EATING GOALS AS JUST ANOTHER REDUCING DIET OR "PROGRAM".**

    Dieting means deprivation, physical and psychological, and almost always assures you will end up fatter and feeling like a failure.

6. KEEP A LOG OF BOTH YOUR EXERCISE AND EATING HABITS.

Keeping a log is a good reinforcer of new habits and can help you in evaluating when or if you need to set different goals.

7. PROGRESS, NOT PERFECTION.

View any lapses, not as failures, but as learning experiences. Focus on what you have done, rather than what you have not done.

8. POSTPONE; DON'T SAY "NO, I CAN'T HAVE IT".

If you forbid yourself to eat a desired food, you will end up obsessing about it and ultimately eat more than would have satisfied you originally. There's a part of us that doesn't want to be told "No".

Instead of saying "No", which almost guarantees you'll eat it anyway, try saying, "I'll wait until after this TV show finishes, and if I still want it, I will have some." Often, you will have forgotten about it by the time the show is over.

9. IF YOUR FRIENDS ARE JEALOUS OF YOUR SUCCESS AND TRY TO SABOTAGE YOU, YOU MAY WISH TO WIDEN YOUR CIRCLE OF ACQUAINTANCES.

Whether or not a person is successful in adopting permanent new habits can be predicted by whether or not they have supportive family and friends. If you are unable to change your family or friends, then learn to be assertive about your own needs. Also learn to tune out harmful (and often well-meant) remarks.

10. WHETHER OR NOT YOU CHANGE YOUR FOOD HABITS, EXERCISE, EXERCISE!

Research shows that people who maintain consistent exercise habits are those most likely to maintain lower body fat levels.

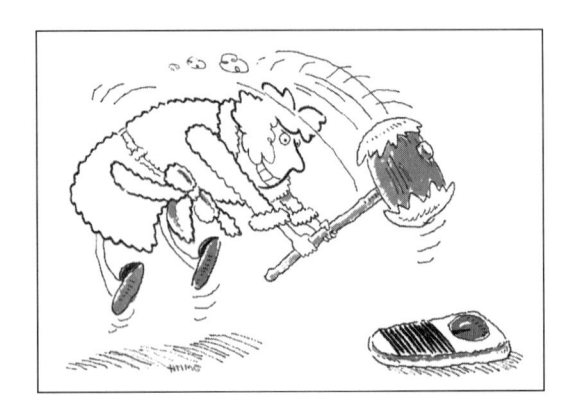

Chapter 15

TABLE OF FOOD VALUES

INTRODUCTION TO THE TABLE OF FOOD VALUES

In case you are wondering what to do with all the information you are about to encounter on the following pages, you can consider it as an aid to your meal planning and grocery shopping. You will notice there are pyramid symbols (▲) in front of many of the food items. We hope this will also assist you in planning healthy meals according to the recommendations outlined on page 35.

▲ indicates that the item is one pyramid serving.
▲▲ indicates that the item is worth two pyramid servings.
▴ indicates 1/2 pyramid serving.

We did not include these symbols on any mixed dishes or the items listed under FRANCHISE RESTAURANTS because the quantities of all the components of these foods were not available to us. Product formulations and nutrition information may change. It is a good idea to check the food label for the most current information.

Obviously, we had to choose which brand name foods to list because the numbers and varieties are endless. If some of your favorite foods or brands are not listed, look at their labels. We attempted to present a representative variety of brand name grocery store foods and menu items from franchise restaurants. Mention of a brand name food or franchise restaurant does not constitute an endorsement or recommendation.

DEFINITION OF TERMS USED ON THE FOOD TABLES

GMS = grams
diam. = diameter
# = pound
?- = no value available
C = cups

oz. = ounce
CALS = calories
NA = sodium
MGS = milligrams

For your convenience in adding figures from the table, fat grams were rounded to the nearest gram. For instance, some tables would show 3.5 gms. of fat. We show 4 gms. instead. Calorie and sodium values were rounded to the nearest 10.

NOTE: The primary source of food values for the calorie, fat and sodium information on the preceding pages was The U.S. Department of Agriculture's Handbook #8, *COMPOSITION OF FOODS*, Nos. 1, 4, 5, 6, 7, 8, 9, 10, 11, 12, 13, 14, 15, 16, 17, 19, 20 and the 1989, 1990, 1991 and 1992 Supplements. Other sources were Pennington, J.A.T. and Church, H.N., Bowes & Church's *FOOD VALUES OF PORTIONS COMMONLY USED*, Sixteenth Edition, 1994, Philadelphia: J.B. Lippincott Company and information from franchise restaurants and the food manufacturing companies.

TABLE OF FOOD VALUES

FOOD	SERVING SIZE	FAT GMS	CALS	NA MGS

STARCHY FOODS: BREAD AND CEREAL PRODUCTS

▲▲= One Pyramid Serving of Bread, Cereal, Pasta and Rice
▲ = One-Half Pyramid Serving of Bread, Cereal, Pasta and Rice

Breads and Bread Products:

Food	Serving Size	Fat	Cals	Na
▲▲Bagel	1 (2 oz.)	1	160	200
Biscuits, From Mix, GOLD MEDAL®:				
▲▲ Biscuit	1 (2.75 in.)	7	160	420
▲▲ Buttermilk Biscuit	1 (2.75 in.)	8	170	420
Biscuits, Refrigerator Dough, PILLSBURY®:				
▲BIG COUNTRY®, Any	1	4	100	300
▲▲Buttermilk, Country	3	3	150	490
▲Bread, Raisin	1 slice	1	70	90
▲Bread, White	1 slice	1	60	120
▲Bread, White, Unsalted	1 slice	1	60	0
▲Bread, Whole Wheat	1 slice	1	60	160
▲Bread, Whole Grain, ROMAN MEAL®	1 slice	1	70	140
▲Breadcrumbs, Dry	1/4 cup	1	100	180
▲Breadsticks, No Salt Coating	3 sticks (1 oz.)	1	120	210
▲▲ Bun, Hamburger	1 bun (1.5 oz.)	2	110	240
▲▲ Bun, Hotdog	1 bun (1.5 oz.)	2	110	240
▲▲Cornbread, From Mix With Egg & Milk	1 piece (2 oz.)	6	180	260
▲Croissant	1 roll (1 oz.)	6	120	170
Crumbs:				
Graham Cracker, SUNSHINE®	3 tablespoons	2	80	150
Plain Bread	1/4 cup	1	100	180
▲▲English Muffin	1 muffin (2 oz.)	1	140	360
Matzo, MANISCHEVITZ®:				
▲Thin, Salted	1 matzo	0	100	120
▲Unsalted	1 matzo	1	110	0
Muffin, From Mix, GOLD MEDAL®:				
▲▲ Basic	1 (3.5 oz.)	8	290	390
▲▲ Blueberry	1 (3.5 oz.)	7	260	320
▲▲ Corn	1 (3.5 oz.)	9	290	570
▲▲ Raisin Bran	1 (3.5 oz.)	8	270	450
Rolls & Bread, Refrigerated, PILLSBURY®:				
▲Breadstick	1 (39 gms.)	3	110	290
▲▲Butterflake Dinner Roll	1	5	130	530
▲▲▲ Crescent	2	11	200	430
Pancakes, Frozen, AUNT JEMINA®:				
▲▲Original	3 cakes	3	200	700
▲▲Buttermilk	3 cakes	3	180	590
▲▲Lowfat	3 cakes	2	130	580
Pancakes, Made From 1/3 C. HUNGRY JACK® Mix With 2% Milk, Oil & Egg:				
▲▲Original	1	13	290	690
▲▲Buttermilk	1	13	290	700
▲▲EXTRA LITE®	1	8	240	630
Pancakes, Made From 1/3 C. HUNGRY JACK® Mix With Skim Milk, Oil & Egg Whites:				
▲▲Original	1	6	220	700
▲▲Buttermilk	1	6	230	710
▲▲EXTRA LITE®	1	6	230	650

Starchy Foods

FOOD	SERVING SIZE	FAT GMS	CALS	NA MGS
Popped Corn Cakes, QUAKER®:				
Popped Corn Cake	2 cakes	0	70	90
Caramel Corn Cake	2 cakes	0	100	110
Rice Cake, Plain	2 cakes	0	70	30
Stuffing Mixes, STOVETOP®:				
▲Beef, Prepared	1/2 cup	9	180	600
▲Chicken, Prepared	1/2 cup	9	170	510
▲Cornbread, Prepared	1/2 cup	8	170	580
▲Long Grain & Wild Rice	1/2 cup	9	180	560
Tortilla:				
▲ Taco Shell, Corn, ROSARITA®	1	2	50	0
▲Tortilla, Corn, Enriched	1 (6" diam.)	1	70	50
Waffle:				
▲▲ Made From Mix With Egg & Milk	1 (7" diam.)	8	210	520
▲NUTRI-GRAIN®, EGGO®, Frozen, Nut and Honey	1 waffle	6	130	250
Cereal Grains and Pasta (Cooked, No Salt Added, Unless Specified Otherwise):				
▲Barley, Pearled	1/2 cup	0	100	0
▲Buckwheat Groats	1/2 cup	1	90	0
▲Bulgur	1/2 cup	0	80	10
▲Corn Grits	1/2 cup	0	70	0
▲Corn Grits, Instant, Plain, QUAKER®	1 packet	0	80	440
Cornmeal, Degermed	1/4 cup	1	130	0
▲Couscous	1/2 cup	0	100	0
▲Farina	1/2 cup	0	60	0
▲Hominy, Canned With Salt	1/2 cup	1	60	170
▲Oat Bran	1/2 cup	1	40	0
Oatmeal:				
▲Regular	1/2 cup	1	70	0
▲Instant, Plain, QUAKER®	1 packet	2	90	270
▲Instant, Maple, QUAKER®	1 packet	2	150	320
▲Quinoa, Raw	2 tablespoons	1	80	?-
Rice:				
▲Brown, Long Grain	1/2 cup	1	110	10
▲White, Long Grain	1/2 cup	0	130	0
▲ Wild	1/2 cup	0	80	0
Rice Mixes, RICE-A-RONI®, Prepared Per Package: (Lower Fat Grams By Omitting Margarine Or Butter Seasoning.)				
Beef Flavor:				
▲▲Regular	1 cup	10	320	1170
▲▲1/3 Less Salt	1 cup	5	280	750
Chicken Flavor:				
▲▲Regular	1 cup	10	320	1100
▲▲1/3 Less Salt	1 cup	5	280	690
▲▲Long Grain & Wild, Original	1 cup	9	290	1240
Rice Mixes, UNCLE BEN'S®, No Fat Added:				
▲▲Fast Cook Long Grain & Wild	1 cup	1	200	850
▲▲Long Grain & Wild Rice Chicken & Herb	3/4 cup	2	200	410
▲▲Long Grain & Wild Rice Vegetable & Herb	3/4 cup	2	200	750
▲▲Natural Long Grain & Wild Rice, Original	1 cup	1	190	63

Starchy Foods

FOOD	SERVING SIZE	FAT GMS	CALS	NA MGS
Pasta, Enriched, Cooked Tender:				
▲Macaroni	1/2 cup	1	100	0
▲Noodles, Egg	1/2 cup	1	110	10
▲Noodles, Spinach	1/2 cup	1	110	10
▲Noodles, Chow Mein	1/2 cup	7	120	100
▲Refrigerator, Plain	2 oz.	1	80	0
▲Refrigerator, Spinach	2 oz.	1	70	0
▲Spaghetti	1/2 cup	1	100	0
▲Spaghetti, Whole Wheat	1/2 cup	0	90	0
Pasta Mixes, NOODLE RONI®, Prepared Per Package: (Lower Fat Grams By Using Skim Milk And Omitting Margarine Or Butter Seasoning.)				
▲▲Angel Hair Pasta With Herbs	1 cup	14	320	840
▲▲Fettuccine Pasta With Broccoli Au Gratin	1 cup	10	290	850
▲▲Oriental Style Pasta With Stir Fry Sauce	1 cup	12	290	1000
Cereals, Ready-To-Eat: (Serving size is 1 ounce unless otherwise stated. Cup measurement varies.)				
GENERAL MILLS®:				
CHEERIOS®:				
▲Honey Nut	1 oz.	2	120	270
▲Plain	1 oz.	2	110	280
▲Multi-Grain	1 oz.	1	110	240
▲CRISPY WHEAT 'N RAISINS®	2 oz.	1	190	270
▲FIBER ONE®	1 oz.	1	60	140
▲GOLDEN GRAHAMS®	1 oz.	1	120	280
▲KIX®	1 oz.	1	120	270
▲TOTAL®	1 oz.	1	110	200
▲TRIPLES®	1 oz.	1	120	190
▲TRIX®	1 oz.	2	120	140
▲WHEATIES®	1 oz.	1	110	220
KELLOGG'S®:				
▲ALL-BRAN®, With Extra Fiber	1/2 cup	1	80	280
▲ALL-BRAN®	1/2 cup	1	50	150
▲APPLE RAISIN CRISP®	1 cup	0	180	340
▲COCOA KRISPIES®	3/4 cup	1	120	190
▲*Common Sense®* Oat Bran With Raisins	1 1/4 cup	3	200	370
▲*Complete®* Bran Flakes	3/4 cup	1	100	230
▲CORNFLAKES®	1 cup	0	110	330
▲CORN POP®	1 cup	0	110	100
▲▲CRACKLIN' OAT BRAN®	3/4 cup (55 gms.)	8	230	180
▲CRISPIX®	1 oz.	0	110	230
▲▲FROSTED MINI-WHEATS®	1 cup (55 gms.)	1	190	0
▲FROSTED FLAKES®	3/4 cup	0	120	200
▲FROOT LOOPS®	1 cup	1	120	150
▲▲FRUITFUL BRAN®	1 1/4 cup (55 gms.)	1	170	330
HEALTHY CHOICE™:				
▲Multi-Grain Flakes	1 cup	0	100	210
▲▲Multi-Grain, Raisins, Crunchy Oat Clusters & Almonds	1 1/4 cup (55 gms.)	2	200	240
▲▲*Just Right®* Fruit & Nut	1 cup (55 gms.)	2	200	250
▲▲Low Fat Granola	1/2 cup (55 gms.)	3	210	120
▲▲*Mueslix®* Golden Crunch	3/4 cup (55 gms.)	5	210	280

Starchy Foods

FOOD	SERVING SIZE	FAT GMS	CALS	NA MGS
KELLOGG'S® (Continued):				
▲Nut & Honey Crunch®	2/3 cup	2	120	200
NUTRI-GRAIN®:				
▲▲Almond Raisin	1 1/4 cup (55 gms.)	3	200	330
▲Golden Wheat	3/4 cup	1	100	240
▲▲Nuggets	1/2 cup (55 gms.)	1	180	350
▲PRODUCT 19®	1 cup	0	110	330
▲▲Raisin Bran	1 cup (55 gms.)	1	170	300
▲Rice Krispies	1 1/4 cup	0	110	360
▲SPECIAL K®	1 cup	0	110	250
MALT-O-MEAL®:				
▲Bran Flakes	3/4 cup	1	100	210
▲Corn Flakes	1 cup	0	110	310
▲Puffed Rice	1 cup	0	60	0
▲Puffed Wheat	1 cup	0	50	0
▲Raisin Bran	1 cup	1	180	260
NABISCO®:				
▲100% Bran	1/3 cup	1	80	120
▲FROSTED WHEAT BITES®	1 cup	1	190	10
▲Shredded Wheat	2 biscuits	1	160	0
▲SHREDDED WHEAT 'N BRAN®	1 1/4 cup	0	200	0
POST®:				
▲ALPHA-BITS®	1 cup	1	130	210
▲BRAN'NOLA® Original	1/2 cup	3	200	240
▲BRAN'NOLA® Raisin	1/2 cup	3	200	220
▲Cocoa PEBBLES®	3/4 cup	1	120	160
▲C.W. POST® Hearty Granola	2/3 cup	9	280	150
▲FRUIT & FIBRE®	1 cup	3	210	260
▲Fruity PEBBLES®	3/4 cup	1	110	150
▲GRAPE-NUTS®	1/2 cup	1	200	350
▲GRAPE-NUTS® Flakes	3/4 cup	1	100	140
▲HONEY BUNCHES OF OATS®	3/4 cup	2	120	190
▲HONEYCOMB®	1 1/3 cup	0	110	190
▲POST TOASTIES®	1 cup	0	100	270
▲Raisin Bran	1 cup	1	190	300
RALSTON®:				
▲Enriched Bran Flakes	1 cup	1	110	220
▲Corn Flakes	1 1/4 cup	0	120	280
▲Corn Chex	1 1/4 cup	0	110	280
▲Double Chex	1 1/4 cup	0	120	230
▲▲Multi-Bran Chex	1 1/4 cup	1	220	300
MUESLI®:				
▲▲ Blueberry Pecan	1 cup	3	200	170
▲▲ Cranberry Walnut	3/4 cup	3	200	180
▲▲ Peach Pecan	3/4 cup	3	200	170
▲▲ Raspberry Almond	3/4 cup	3	220	170
▲▲ Strawberry Pecan	1 cup	3	210	170
▲▲ Raisin Bran	3/4 cup	1	190	280
▲Rice Chex	1 cup	0	120	230
▲Sun Flakes	3/4 cup	1	110	210
▲▲ Wheat Chex	3/4 cup	1	190	390
Crackers:				
KEEBLER®:				
▲HONEY GRAHAM SELECTS®	8 crackers	6	150	140
▲Low Fat CINNAMON CRISP®	8 crackers	2	110	190
▲Low Fat Honey Graham	9 crackers	2	120	210
▲MUNCH'EMS®, Ranch	28 crackers	5	130	340

Starchy Foods

FOOD	SERVING SIZE	FAT GMS	CALS	NA MGS
Crackers (Continued):				
KEEBLER® (Continued):				
▲MUNCH'EMS®, Salsa, Lowfat	28 crackers	4	140	260
▲WHEATABLES®, Original	26 crackers	7	150	320
▲WHEATABLES®, Ranch	25 crackers	7	150	310
▲WHEATABLES®, Reduced Sodium	25 crackers	7	150	160
▲WHEATABLES®, Reduced Fat	29 crackers	4	130	320
NABISCO®:				
▲BETTER CHEDDARS®, Regular	22 crackers	8	150	290
▲BETTER CHEDDARS®, Reduced Fat	24 crackers	6	140	350
▲HARVEST CRISPS®, 5-Grain	13 crackers	4	130	300
▲ OYSTERETTES®	19 crackers	3	60	150
▲ PREMIUM®, Original	5 crackers	2	60	180
▲ PREMIUM®, Fat Free	5 crackers	0	50	130
▲ RITZ®, Regular	5 crackers	4	80	140
▲ RITZ®, Reduced Fat	5 crackers	3	70	140
▲ SNACKWELL'S® Cracked Pepper	7 crackers	0	60	150
▲TRISCUIT®, Regular	7 crackers	5	140	170
▲TRISCUIT®, Reduced Fat	8 crackers	3	130	180
▲ WAVERLY®	5 crackers	4	70	140
▲WHEAT THINS®, Regular	16 crackers	6	140	170
▲WHEAT THINS®, Reduced Fat	18 crackers	4	120	220
▲WHEAT THINS®, Multi Grain	17 crackers	4	130	290
RALSTON-PURINA®:				
▲ RY-KRISP®, Original	2 crackers	0	60	80
▲ RY-KRISP®, Seasoned	2 crackers	2	60	90
▲ RY-KRISP®, Sesame	2 crackers	2	60	80
▲ WHEAT KRISP®	2 crackers	2	70	150
SUNSHINE®:				
▲Animal Crackers	14 crackers	4	140	130
▲CHEEZ-IT®	27 crackers	8	160	240
▲CHEEZ-IT® Hot & Spicy	26 crackers	8	160	220
▲CHEEZ-IT®, Low Sodium	27 crackers	8	160	70
▲CHEEZ-IT® White Cheddar	26 crackers	9	160	280
▲Grahams, Cinnamon	2 crackers	6	140	150
▲Grahams, Honey	2 crackers	4	120	130
▲HI HO®	9 crackers	9	160	280
▲HI HO® Butter Flavor	9 crackers	9	160	280
▲HI HO® Cracked Pepper	9 crackers	9	160	280
▲HI HO® Multi Grain	9 crackers	9	160	370
▲HI HO® Reduced Fat	10 crackers	5	140	280
▲HI HO® Whole Wheat	9 crackers	8	150	280
▲ KRISPY® Cracked Pepper	5 crackers	2	60	180
▲ KRISPY® Original	5 crackers	2	60	180
▲ KRISPY® Unsalted Tops	5 crackers	2	60	120
▲ KRISPY® Soup & Oyster	17 crackers	2	60	200
▲ KRISPY® Whole Wheat	5 crackers	2	60	130
Flour:				
Rice, White	1/2 cup	1	290	0
Wheat, All Purpose	1/2 cup	1	230	0
Wheat, Whole Wheat	1/2 cup	1	200	0
Tapioca, Minute, Dry	1 tablespoon	0	30	0
Wheat Germ, Toasted	2 tablespoons	3	50	0
Wheat Bran, Toasted	1/3 cup	2	60	0

FOOD	SERVING SIZE	FAT GMS	CALS	NA MGS

FRUITS AND FRUIT JUICES

▲ = One Pyramid Serving Of Fruits

Apple:

▲Raw With Skin	1 (3" diam.)	1	80	0
▲▲Dried, Uncooked	1/2 cup	0	100	40
▲Apple Juice	3/4 cup	0	90	10

Applesauce, Canned:

▲Unsweetened	1/2 cup	0	50	0
▲Sweetened	1/2 cup	0	100	0

Apricots:

▲Raw	1/2 cup halves	0	40	0
Canned:				
▲Juice Pack	1/2 cup halves	0	60	10
▲Syrup Pack, Heavy	1/2 cup halves	0	110	10
▲Syrup Pack, Lite	1/2 cup halves	0	80	10
▲▲Dried, Uncooked	1/2 cup halves	0	190	10
▲Apricot Nectar, Canned	3/4 cup	0	110	10
▲Avocado	1/2	15	160	10
▲Banana	1 medium (9" long)	1	110	0
▲▲Blackberries, Raw	1 cup	1	70	0
▲▲Blueberries, Raw	1 cup	1	80	10
▲▲Cantaloupe	1/2 (5" diam.)	1	90	20

Cherries:

▲Sweet, Raw	1/2 cup	1	50	0
Canned:				
▲Sweet, Juice Pack	1/2 cup	0	70	0
▲Sweet, Syrup Pack, Heavy	1/2 cup	0	110	0
▲Frozen, Sweetened	1/2 cup	0	120	0

Cranberries:

Raw, Whole	1/2 cup	0	20	0
▲ Sauce, Canned, Sweetened	1/4 cup	0	110	20
▲Cranberry Juice Cocktail, Sweetened	3/4 cup	0	110	10
▲Currants, Dried	1/4 cup	0	100	0
▲Dates	1/4 cup	0	120	0

Figs:

▲Raw	1 large	0	50	0
Canned:				
▲Syrup Pack, Heavy	1/2 cup	0	110	0
▲Syrup Pack, Light	1/2 cup	0	90	0
▲Dried, Uncooked	1/4 cup	1	130	10

Fruit Cocktail, Canned:

▲Juice Pack	1/2 cup	0	60	0
▲Syrup Pack, Heavy	1/2 cup	0	90	10

Grapefruit:

▲Raw	1/2 (4" diam.)	0	40	0
Canned:				
▲Juice Pack	1/2 cup	0	50	10
▲Syrup Pack, Light	1/2 cup	0	80	0

Grapefruit Juice, Unsweetened:

▲Canned	3/4 cup	0	70	0
▲Frozen, Diluted (3:1)	3/4 cup	0	80	0

Fruits and Fruit Juices

FOOD	SERVING SIZE	FAT GMS	CALS	NA MGS
Grapes:				
Raw:				
▲▲Slip Skin	1 cup	0	60	0
▲▲SeedlessSkin	1 cup	1	100	0
▲Canned,				
Syrup Pack, Heavy	1/2 cup	0	90	10
Grape Juice:				
▲Canned Or Bottled	3/4 cup	0	120	10
▲Frozen, Diluted (3:1)	3/4 cup	0	100	0
▲Honeydew Melon	1 wedge (7" x 2")	0	50	10
▲Kiwifruit	1 medium	0	50	0
Lemon Or Lime Juice	1/2 cup	0	30	0
Lemon Or Lime Juice	1 tablespoon	0	0	0
▲Mangos, Raw	1/2 cup slices	0	50	0
▲Nectarines	1 (2.5" diam.)	1	70	0
Oranges:				
▲Raw	1 (2.5" diam.)	0	60	0
▲Mandarin, Canned, Light Syrup	1/2 cup	0	80	10
▲Orange Juice, Frozen, Diluted (3:1)	3/4 cup	0	80	0
▲Papaya, Raw	1 fruit	0	120	10
Peaches:				
▲Raw	1 (2.5" diam.)	0	40	0
Canned:				
▲Juice Pack	1/2 cup	0	60	10
▲Syrup Pack, Heavy	1/2 cup	0	100	10
▲Dried, Uncooked	1/4 cup	0	90	0
▲Frozen, Sliced, Sweetened	1/2 cup	0	120	10
▲Peach Nectar, Canned	3/4 cup	0	100	10
Pears:				
▲Raw, Bartlett	1 (2.5" x 3.5")	1	100	0
Canned:				
▲Juice Pack	1/2 cup	0	60	10
▲Syrup Pack, Heavy	1/2 cup	0	90	10
▲Dried, Uncooked	1/4 cup	0	120	0
▲Pear Nectar, Canned	3/4 cup	0	110	0
Pineapple:				
▲Raw	1/2 cup diced	0	40	0
Canned:				
▲Juice Pack	1/2 cup	0	80	0
▲Syrup Pack	1/2 cup	0	100	0
▲Pineapple Juice, Canned	3/4 cup	0	100	0
▲Plantain, Cooked	1/2 cup sliced	0	90	0
Plums:				
▲Raw	1 (2" diam.)	0	40	0
Canned:				
▲Juice Pack	1/2 cup	0	70	0
▲Syrup Pack, Heavy	1/2 cup	0	120	30
Prunes:				
▲Canned, Syrup Pack	1/2 cup	0	120	0
▲▲Dried, Uncooked	1/2 cup	0	190	0
▲Prune Juice, Canned	3/4 cup	0	140	10
▲Raisins, Seedless	1/4 cup packed	0	110	0
Raspberries:				
▲▲Raw	1 cup	1	60	0
▲Frozen, Sweetened	1/2 cup	0	130	0

Fruits and Fruit Juices

FOOD	SERVING SIZE	FAT GMS	CALS	NA MGS
Rhubarb:				
▲Raw	1/2 cup diced	0	10	0
▲Frozen, Sweetened	1/2 cup	0	140	0
Strawberries:				
▲▲Raw	1 cup	1	50	0
▲Frozen, Sweetened	1/2 cup slices	0	120	0
▲Tangerines	1 (2.5" diam.)	0	40	0
▲▲Watermelon	1 slice (10"x1")	2	150	10

VEGETABLES, COOKED WITHOUT FAT, SAUCES OR OTHER INGREDIENTS, UNLESS SPECIFIED OTHERWISE

▲ = One Pyramid Serving of Vegetables
▲ = One-Half Pyramid Serving of Vegetables

FOOD	SERVING SIZE	FAT GMS	CALS	NA MGS
▲Arugula, Raw	1 cup	0	0	10
▲Alfalfa Sprouts, Raw	1/2 cup	0	10	0
▲Artichoke Hearts	1/2 cup	0	40	80
Asparagus:				
▲Fresh, Cooked	1/2 cup	0	20	10
▲Canned	1/2 cup	0	20	430
Bamboo Shoots:				
▲Raw	1/2 cup	0	10	0
▲Canned	1/2 cup	0	10	10
▲Beans, Snap (Italian, Green Or Yellow), Fresh, Cooked	1/2 cup	0	20	10
Beans, All Others (See Legumes)				
Beets:				
▲Fresh, Cooked	1/2 cup slices	0	30	40
▲Canned	1/2 cup slices	0	40	320
▲Harvard, Canned	1/2 cup slices	0	90	200
▲Pickled, Canned	1/2 cup slices	0	80	300
▲Greens, Fresh, Cooked	1/2 cup	0	20	170
Broccoli:				
▲Raw	1/2 cup chopped	0	10	10
▲Fresh, Cooked	1/2 cup	0	20	20
Frozen, Cheese Sauce:				
▲BIRD'S EYE®	1/2 cup	6	120	490
▲GREEN GIANT®	2/3 cup	3	70	520
▲Frozen, Cooked, Plain	1/2 cup chopped	0	30	20
Brussels Sprouts:				
▲Fresh Or Frozen, Cooked	1/2 cup	0	30	20
▲Frozen, Cheese Sauce, BIRD'S EYE®	1/2 cup	6	110	420
Cabbage, Shredded:				
▲Raw	1/2 cup	0	10	10
▲Fresh, Cooked	1/2 cup	0	20	10
▲Chinese, Raw	1/2 cup	0	10	20
▲Chinese, Fresh, Cooked	1/2 cup	0	10	30
▲Coleslaw, Homemade Cream Style Dressing	1/2 cup	2	40	10
Carrots:				
▲Baby, Raw	10 (approx. 3")	1	40	30
▲Raw	1 (approx. 7")	0	30	30
▲Carrot Raisin Salad	1/2 cup			
▲Fresh, Cooked	1/2 cup slices	0	40	50
▲Juice, Canned	3/4 cup	0	80	50

Fruits, Fruit Juices and Vegetables 71

FOOD	SERVING SIZE	FAT GMS	CALS	NA MGS
Cauliflower:				
▲Raw	1/2 cup (1" pieces)	0	20	10
▲Fresh, Cooked	1/2 cup	0	20	10
▲Frozen, Cheese Sauce, BIRD'S EYE®	1/2 cup	6	110	480
Celery:				
▲Raw	1/2 cup diced	0	10	50
▲Stalk, Raw	2	0	10	70
▲Fresh, Cooked	1/2 cup diced	0	10	70
▲Chard, Swiss, Fresh, Cooked	1/2 cup chopped	0	20	160
Chives	Any amount	0	0	0
▲Collards	1/2 cup chopped	0	20	10
Corn:				
Kernels, Fresh, Cooked	1/2 cup or 1/2 ear	0	70	0
Canned:				
▲Plain	1/2 cup	1	80	320
▲Cream Style	1/2 cup	1	90	370
▲Cucumber, Raw	1/2 cup slices	0	10	0
▲Dandelion Greens, Fresh, Cooked	1/2 cup	0	20	20
▲Eggplant, Fresh, Cooked	1/2 cup cubed	0	10	0
▲Endive, Raw	1 cup chopped	0	10	10
▲Hominy, White	1/2 cup	1	60	170
▲Jerusalem-Artichoke, Raw	1/2 cup slices	0	60	?-
▲Kale, Raw	1 cup chopped	0	30	30
▲Kale, Fresh, Cooked	1/2 cup	0	20	20
▲Kohlrabi	1/2 cup slices	0	20	20
▲Leek, Raw	1/2 cup chopped	0	30	10
Legumes (Also see PROTEIN FOODS):				
▲▲Beans, Baked, Homemade	1 cup	13	380	1070
Beans, Canned:				
▲▲Black	1 cup	1	220	920
▲▲Black, Refried, OLD EL PASO®	1 cup	4	240	680
▲▲Chili, Mexican Style	1 cup	2	210	730
▲▲Cow-Peas/Crowder	1 cup	1	180	720
▲▲Garbanzo/Chickpeas	1 cup	3	290	720
▲▲Great Northern, Unsalted	1 cup	1	300	10
▲▲Kidney	1 cup	1	220	870
▲▲Lima	1 cup	0	190	810
▲▲Navy	1 cup	1	300	1170
▲▲Pinto	1 cup	1	190	1000
▲▲Pork/Tomato Sauce	1 cup	3	250	1110
▲▲Refried	1 cup	4	240	760
▲▲Refried, Fat Free, OLD EL PASO®	1 cup	0	220	960
▲▲Three Bean Salad	1 cup	1	180	1480
▲With Franks	1 cup	17	370	1110
▲▲White	1 cup	1	250	1190
Beans, Dry, Most Varieties, Not Canned:				
▲▲Lentils, Boiled	1 cup	1	230	0
Lima, Boiled:				
▲▲Fresh	1 cup	1	210	30
▲▲Baby, Frozen	1 cup	1	190	50
▲▲Fordhook, Frozen	1 cup	1	170	90
▲▲Split Peas, Boiled	1 cup	1	230	0
▲White Beans, Boiled	1 cup	1	250	10

Vegetables

FOOD	SERVING SIZE	FAT GMS	CALS	NA MGS
Bean Products:				
▲Falafel	3 patties	9	170	150
▲Hummus, Homemade	1/2 cup	10	210	30
Soybeans And Products:				
▲Boiled, Plain	1/2 cup	8	150	0
▲Roasted, Dry	1/4 cup	9	190	0
Miso	1/2 cup	8	280	5030
Natto	1/2 cup	10	190	10
▲Soy Milk (Use as Milk Substitute)	1 cup	5	80	30
Tempeh	1/2 cup	6	170	10
Tofu (Soybean Curd):				
▲Raw, Firm	1/2 cup	11	180	20
▲Raw, Regular	1/2 cup	6	90	10
▲Sprouts, Mung, Raw	1/2 cup	0	20	0
Lettuce, Raw:				
▲Boston & Bibb Types	1 head	0	20	10
▲Iceberg	1/4 head	0	20	10
▲Looseleaf	1 cup shredded	0	10	10
▲Romaine	1 cup shredded	0	10	0
Mushrooms:				
▲Raw	1/2 cup slices	0	10	0
▲Canned	1/2 cup pieces	0	20	?-
▲Fresh, Cooked	1/2 cup pieces	0	20	0
▲Shiitake, Dried, Cooked	1/2 cup	0	40	0
▲Mustard Greens, Fresh, Cooked	1/2 cup chopped	0	10	10
▲New Zealand Spinach, Fresh, Cooked	1/2 cup chopped	0	10	100
▲Okra, Frozen, Cooked	1/2 cup slices	0	30	0
Onions:				
▲Raw	1/2 cup chopped	0	30	0
▲Fresh, Cooked	1/2 cup chopped	0	50	0
▲Rings, Frozen, Prepared In Oven	7 rings	19	290	260
▲Canned	1/2 cup	0	20	420
▲Green, Raw	1/2 chopped	0	20	10
▲Parsley, Raw	1 cup chopped	0	20	30
▲Parsnips, Fresh, Cooked	1/2 cup slices	0	60	10
Peas, Edible-Pods:				
▲Fresh, Cooked	1/2 cup	0	30	0
▲Frozen, Cooked	1/2 cup	0	40	0
Peas, Green:				
▲Fresh, Cooked	1/2 cup	0	70	0
▲Canned	1/2 cup	0	60	190
▲Frozen, Cooked	1/2 cup	0	60	70
▲With Carrots, Canned	1/2 cup	0	50	330
▲With Carrots, Frozen, Cooked	1/2 cup	0	40	60
▲With Onions, Frozen, Cooked	1/2 cup	0	40	?-
Peppers, Green Or Red:				
▲Raw	1/2 cup chopped	0	20	0
▲Canned	1/2 cup halves	0	10	960
▲Hot Chili	1/2 cup	0	20	?-
▲Poi	1/2 cup	0	130	10

Vegetables

FOOD	SERVING SIZE	FAT GMS	CALS	NA MGS
Potatoes:				
▲Au Gratin, Homemade	1/2 cup	9	160	530
▲Au Gratin, From Dry Mix	1/2 cup	6	130	600
▲Baked With Skin	1 (approx. 7 oz.)	2	220	20
▲Baked Without Skin	1/2 cup	0	60	0
▲Boiled	1/2 cup	0	70	0
▲Canned	1/2 cup	0	50	?-
Chips (See Snack Foods On Page 91):				
▲From Dehydrated Flakes, With Milk & Salt	1/2 cup	6	120	350
▲French-Fried, Heated In Oven, Home	10 strips	4	110	20
▲Fried In Oil, Restaurant	10 strips	8	160	110
▲Hashed Brown In Fat	1/2 cup	11	160	20
▲Mashed With Whole Milk & Fat, Salt Added	1/2 cup	4	110	310
▲Scalloped, Homemade	1/2 cup	5	110	410
▲Scalloped, From Dry Mix, With Milk & Fat	1/2 cup	6	130	470
▲Salad	1/2 cup	10	180	660
▲Sticks	1/2 cup	6	90	50
▲Sweet, Baked	1/2 cup mashed	0	100	10
▲Sweet, Canned, Syrup Pack	1/2 cup	0	110	40
▲Tater Tots, ORE IDA®	3 ounces	7	150	400
▲Pumpkin, Canned	1/2 cup	0	40	10
▲Radicchio, Raw	1 cup shredded	0	10	10
▲Radishes, Raw	13	0	10	10
▲Rutabagas, Fresh, Cooked	1/2 cup mashed	0	40	20
▲Sauerkraut, Canned	1/2 cup	0	20	780
Spinach:				
▲Raw	1 cup chopped	0	10	40
▲Canned	1/2 cup	0	20	370
▲Fresh, Cooked	1/2 cup	0	20	60
▲Frozen, Cooked	1/2 cup	0	30	80
▲Frozen, Cream Style, GREEN GIANT®	1/2 cup	3	80	520
▲ Souffle, Homemade	1 cup	18	220	760
Squash:				
▲Raw	1/2 cup slices	0	10	0
▲Summer, Fresh, Cooked	1/2 cup slices	0	20	0
▲Winter, Baked	1/2 cup cubes	1	40	0
Tomatoes:				
▲Green, Raw	1 (approx. 2.5")	0	30	20
▲Red, Ripe, Raw	1 (approx. 2.5")	0	30	10
Canned:				
▲Juice	3/4 cup	0	30	660
▲Paste, Unsalted	1/4 cup	1	60	40
▲Pureed, Unsalted	1/2 cup	0	50	30
▲Red, Ripe, Whole	1/2 cup	0	20	200
▲Sauce, Salted	1/2 cup	0	40	740
▲Stewed	1/2 cup	0	30	330
Catsup	1 tablespoon	0	20	180
▲Sun-Dried	1/4 cup	0	40	280

Vegetables

FOOD	SERVING SIZE	FAT GMS	CALS	NA MGS
Spaghetti Sauce, Canned:				
▲Marinara	1/2 cup	4	90	1290
▲HUNT'S® Traditional	1/2 cup	2	70	530
▲PREGO®, Traditional	1/2 cup	6	150	640
▲PREGO®, Garden Harvest Light	1/2 cup	0	50	390
▲RAGU®, Traditional	1/2 cup	4	80	820
▲RAGU®, Spicy Red Pepper	1/2 cup	2	100	530
▲RAGU®, Tomato & Herb, Light	1/2 cup	0	50	390
Turnips:				
▲Raw	1/2 cup cubes	0	20	40
▲Fresh, Cooked	1/2 cup cubes	0	10	40
▲Greens, Fresh, Cooked	1/2 cup chopped	0	20	20
▲Greens, Canned	1/2 cup	0	20	330
▲Vegetable Juice Cocktail	3/4 cup	0	30	660
Vegetables, Mixed:				
▲Canned	1/2 cup	0	40	120
▲Frozen	1/2 cup	0	50	30
▲Waterchestnuts, Canned	1/2 cup slices	0	40	10
▲Watercress, Raw	1 cup chopped	0	0	10

DAIRY PRODUCTS
▲ = One Pyramid Serving of Milk, Yogurt or Cheese
▲ = One-Half Pyramid Serving of Milk, Yogurt or Cheese

Cheeses:				
▲American Pasteurized Process Cheese	2 oz.	18	220	810
▲Blue	1.5 oz.	12	150	590
▲Brie	1.5 oz.	12	140	270
▲Camembert	1.5 oz.	10	130	360
▲Cheddar	1.5 oz.	14	170	260
▲Colby	1.5 oz.	14	170	260
Cottage Cheese:				
Creamed	1/2 cup	5	110	430
2% Fat	1/2 cup	2	100	460
1% Fat	1/2 cup	1	80	460
Cream Cheese	2 tablespoons	10	100	80
▲Edam	1.5 oz.	12	150	410
▲Feta	1.5 oz.	9	120	470
▲Goat, Semi-Soft	1.5 oz.	12	150	220
▲Goat, Soft	1.5 oz.	9	120	160
▲Gouda	1.5 oz	12	150	350
▲Gruyere	1.5 oz.	14	180	140
▲Monterey	1.5 oz.	14	170	230
▲Mozzarella, Low Moisture Part Skim Milk	2 oz.	10	160	300
▲Muenster	1.5 oz.	14	150	270
Parmesan, Grated	2 tablespoons	3	50	190
▲Provolone	1.5 oz.	12	150	370
Ricotta, Part Skim Milk	1/2 cup	10	170	160
Romano	1 oz.	8	110	340
▲Roquefort	1.5 oz.	14	170	770
Swiss:				
▲Natural	1.5 oz.	12	170	110
▲Pasteurized Process	2 oz.	14	200	780

Vegetables and Dairy Products

FOOD	SERVING SIZE	FAT GMS	CALS	NA MGS
KRAFT® Brand, Various Types:				
▲ KRAFT FREE® Singles, Nonfat Pasteurized	1 slice (.6 oz.)	0	30	290
▲ Cheddar, Sharp, Lowfat	1 oz.	5	80	210
▲ CHEEZ WHIZ® Squeezable Sauce	2 tablespoons	8	100	470
▲ CHEEZ WHIZ® LIGHT	2 tablespoons	3	80	540
▲ CRACKER BARREL® Sharp Cheddar Cold Pack Cheese Food	2 tablespoons	8	100	290
100% Grated Romano	2 teaspoons	2	30	90
▲ String Cheese, Low Moisture	1 oz.	6	80	240
▲ VELVEETA® Pasteurized Process Cheese Spread	1 oz.	6	80	420
▲ VELVEETA® LIGHT	1 oz.	3	60	420
KRAFT HEALTHY FAVORITES®:				
▲ Cheddar, Fat Free	1/4 cup shredded	0	50	220
▲ Mozzarella, Fat Free	1/4 cup shredded	0	50	280
PHILADELPHIA BRAND® Cream Cheese:				
▲ FREE®	2 tablespoons soft	0	30	160
▲ LIGHT®	2 tablespoons soft	5	70	150
NEUFCHATEL®	2 tablespoons soft	6	70	120
▲ Regular	2 tablespoons soft	10	100	100
SPREADERY® Cheese Snack NEUFCHATEL®:				
▲ Classic Ranch	2 tablespoons	7	80	210
▲ Garden Vegetables	2 tablespoons	6	70	230
▲ Garlic & Herb	2 tablespoons	7	80	180
Cream:				
Half 'N Half	2 tablespoons	3	40	10
Sour	2 tablespoons	5	50	10
Sour, SEALTEST®	2 tablespoons	5	60	20
Sour, Fat Free, SEALTEST®	2 tablespoons	0	40	30
Sour, Light, SEALTEST®	2 tablespoons	3	40	20
Whipping, Heavy, Fluid	2 tablespoons	11	100	10
Whipped Cream, Canned, Pressurized	2 tablespoons	1	20	10
Cream Substitute:				
Frozen, Liquid	2 tablespoons	3	40	20
Powdered	1 tablespoon	2	30	10
Milk, Cow's:				
▲Buttermilk, Cultured	1 cup	2	100	260
Chocolate:				
▲Whole	1 cup	8	210	150
▲2% Fat	1 cup	5	180	150
▲1% Fat	1 cup	3	160	150
Canned:				
Condensed, Sweet	1 cup	27	980	390
▲Evaporated Skim	1/2 cup	0	100	150
▲Evaporated Whole	1/2 cup	10	170	130
▲Lowfat, 2%	1 cup	5	120	120
▲Lowfat, 1%	1 cup	3	100	120
▲Skim, With Nonfat Milk Solids Added	1 cup	1	90	130
▲Whole, 3.3% Fat	1 cup	8	150	120
▲Milkshake, Vanilla	11 oz.	10	350	300

Dairy Products

FOOD	SERVING SIZE	FAT GMS	CALS	NA MGS
▲Milk, Goat's	1 cup	10	170	120
Yogurt:				
▲Plain	1 cup	7	140	110
Lowfat:				
▲Coffee And Vanilla	1 cup	3	190	150
▲Fruit Flavors	1 cup	3	230	120
▲Plain	1 cup	4	140	160
▲Nonfat, Plain	1 cup	0	130	170

PROTEIN FOODS: LEGUMES, MEAT, FISH, POULTRY AND EGGS

▲ = One Pyramid Serving of Dried Beans, Nuts, Meat, Fish, Poultry and Eggs
▴ = One-half Pyramid Serving of Dried Beans, Nuts, Meat, Fish, Poultry and Eggs

FOOD	SERVING SIZE	FAT GMS	CALS	NA MGS
Beef, Cooked:				
▲Breakfast Strips	3 strips	12	150	770
▲DELI THIN®, OSCAR MAYER®, Roast Beef	2 oz.	2	60	530
Brisket, Braised:				
▲Corned Beef	3 oz.	16	210	960
▲Flat, Fat & Lean	2 oz.	16	210	30
▲Flat, Lean Only	2 oz.	4	110	40
▲Point Half, Lean Only	2 oz.	8	140	40
Chuck, Pot Roast:				
▲Arm, Lean Only	2 oz.	5	120	40
▲Blade, Lean Only	2 oz.	8	140	40
▲Dried, Chipped	2 oz.	2	90	1970
▲Flank Steak, Lean & Fat	2 oz.	9	150	40
▲Flank Steak, Lean Only	2 oz.	7	140	40
Ground:				
▲Extra Lean	2 oz.	9	150	40
▲Lean	2 oz.	11	160	40
▲Regular	2 oz.	13	180	50
Rib:				
Prime Rib, Roasted:				
▲Fat & Lean	2 oz.	20	230	40
▲Lean Only	2 oz.	11	170	40
Rib Eye, Broiled:				
▲Fat & Lean	2 oz.	13	180	40
▲Lean Only	2 oz.	7	130	40
▲Short Ribs, Fat & Lean	2 oz.	24	270	30
Steaks, Lean & Fat, Broiled:				
▲Porterhouse	2 oz.	13	170	40
▴T-Bone	2 oz.	12	170	40
Steaks, Lean Only:				
▲Porterhouse/T-Bone, Broiled	2 oz.	6	120	40
▲Round Steak, Bottom, Braised	2 oz.	2	110	30
Tenderloin, Lean & Fat:				
▲Broiled	2 oz.	12	170	30
▲Roasted	2 oz.	15	190	30
Tenderloin, Lean Only:				
▲Broiled	2 oz.	5	120	40
▲Roasted	2 oz.	7	130	40
Egg, Boiled Or Poached:				
▴ Whole	1 large	5	80	60
▴ White	2	0	30	110
▴ Egg, Fried, Salted	1 large	7	90	160

Dairy Products and Protein Foods

FOOD	SERVING SIZE	FAT GMS	CALS	NA MGS
Egg Substitutes:				
▲ EGG BEATERS®	1/4 cup	0	30	80
▲ SCRAMBLERS®	1/4 cup	2	60	90
Fish, Baked Or Broiled:				
▲Bass, Freshwater	3 oz.	4	120	80
▲Bass, Striped	3 oz.	3	110	80
▲Bluefish	3 oz.	5	140	70
▲Carp	3 oz.	6	140	50
▲Cod	3 oz.	1	90	70
▲Dolphinfish	3 oz.	1	90	100
▲Eel	3 oz.	13	200	60
▲Flounder Or Sole	3 oz.	1	100	90
▲Grouper	3 oz.	1	100	50
▲Haddock	3 oz.	1	100	70
▲Halibut	3 oz.	3	120	60
▲Herring	3 oz.	10	170	100
▲Mackerel	3 oz.	15	220	70
▲Monkfish	3 oz.	2	80	20
▲Perch (Redfish)	3 oz.	2	100	80
▲Pike, Northern	3 oz.	1	100	40
▲Pike, Walleye	3 oz.	1	100	60
▲Pollock	3 oz.	1	100	90
▲Pompano	3 oz.	10	180	70
▲Roughy, Orange	3 oz.	1	80	70
▲Salmon, Atlantic	3 oz.	7	160	50
▲Seabass	3 oz.	2	110	70
▲Snapper	3 oz.	2	110	50
▲Sturgeon	3 oz.	4	120	?
▲Swordfish	3 oz.	4	130	100
▲Trout, Mixed Species	3 oz.	7	160	60
▲Tuna, Yellow Fin	3 oz.	1	120	40
▲Turbot	3 oz.	3	100	160
▲Whitefish	3 oz.	6	150	60
▲Whiting	3 oz.	1	100	110
Fish, Canned:				
Anchovies, Drained	5 anchovies	2	180	730
▲Clams, Drained	3 oz.	2	130	?-
▲Gefilte Fish	2 pieces (approx. 3 oz.)	2	70	440
▲Mackerel, Drained	1/4 can (#300)	6	140	340
Salmon:				
▲Pink With Bone	3 oz.	5	120	470
▲Red With Bone	3 oz.	6	130	460
▲ Sardines, Drained	3 sardines	4	80	180
Tuna, Drained:				
▲▲In Oil	1 can (6.5 oz.)	14	330	700
▲▲In Water	1 can (6.5 oz.)	5	220	650
▲Crab, Drained	3 oz.	1	80	280
▲Shrimp	3 oz.	2	100	140
▲Clams, Drained	3 oz.	2	130	?-
▲ Oysters, Solids & Liquids	3 oz.	2	60	?-
Fish, Miscellaneous:				
▲Catfish, Channel, Breaded, Fried	3 oz.	11	190	240
▲ Caviar, Black & Red	2 tablespoons	6	80	480
▲Cod, Dried, Salted	1 oz.	1	80	1970
▲Croaker, Breaded, Fried	3 oz.	11	190	300
▲ Fish Cakes, Fillets, Sticks, Frozen, Breaded, Fried	2 oz.	7	160	330

Protein Foods

FOOD	SERVING SIZE	FAT GMS	CALS	NA MGS
Fish, Miscellaneous (Continued):				
Herring:				
▲ Kippered	2 oz.	7	120	510
Pickled	1 oz.	5	80	260
▲Salmon, Smoked	3 oz.	4	100	670
▲Shark, Batter-Dipped, Fried	3 oz.	12	190	100
▲Surimi	3 oz.	1	80	120
▲ Tuna Salad	1/2 cup	10	190	410
Shellfish:				
Crab:				
▲ Cakes, Fried	2 pcs.	5	90	200
▲Dungeness, Boiled	3 oz.	1	90	320
▲Imitation	3 oz.	1	90	720
▲Crayfish, Boiled	3 oz.	1	100	60
▲Lobster, Boiled	3 oz.	1	80	320
Shrimp:				
▲Boiled	3 oz.	1	80	190
▲Breaded, Fried	3 oz.	10	210	290
▲Imitation	3 oz.	1	90	600
Mollusks:				
▲Abalone, Breaded, Fried	3 oz.	6	160	500
Clams:				
▲Breaded, Fried	3 oz.	10	170	310
▲Steamed	3 oz.	2	130	100
▲Mussels, Steamed	3 oz.	4	150	310
▲Octopus, Boiled	3 oz.	2	140	?-
Oysters:				
▲ Breaded, Fried	6 medium	11	170	360
▲Raw, Eastern	12 medium	4	120	190
▲Steamed	3 oz.	4	120	190
Scallops:				
▲Breaded, Fried	6 large	10	200	430
▲Imitation	3 oz.	0	80	680
▲Raw	3 oz.	1	80	140
▲Squid, Fried	3 oz.	6	150	260
Game, Roasted:				
▲Beefalo	3 oz.	5	160	70
▲Bison	3 oz.	2	120	50
▲Deer	3 oz.	3	130	50
▲Elk	3 oz.	2	120	50
▲Goat	3 oz.	3	120	70
▲Moose	3 oz.	1	110	60
▲Rabbit, Domesticated	3 oz.	7	170	40
▲Rabbit, Wild	3 oz.	3	150	40
▲Squirrel	3 oz.	4	150	100
Lamb, Lean:				
Arm And Blade, Braised:				
▲Lean & Fat	3 oz.	21	290	60
▲Lean Only	3 oz.	14	240	70
▲Leg, Lean Only	3 oz.	6	150	60
▲Loin Chop, Lean Only, Broiled	3 oz.	8	190	70
▲Loin, Lean & Fat, Roasted	3 oz.	20	270	60

Protein Foods

FOOD	SERVING SIZE	FAT GMS	CALS	NA MGS
Legumes:				
▲Beans, Baked, Homemade	1 cup	13	380	1070
Beans, Canned:				
▲Black	1 cup	1	220	920
▲Chili, Mexican Style	1 cup	2	210	730
▲Cow-Peas/Crowder	1 cup	1	180	720
▲Garbanzo/Chickpeas	1 cup	3	290	720
▲Great Northern, Unsalted	1 cup	1	300	10
▲Kidney	1 cup	1	220	870
▲Lima	1 cup	0	190	810
▲Navy	1 cup	1	300	1170
▲Pinto	1 cup	1	190	1000
▲Pork/Tomato Sauce	1 cup	3	250	1110
▲Refried	1 cup	4	240	760
▲ Three Bean Salad	1 cup	1	180	1480
▲With Franks	1 cup	17	370	1110
▲White	1 cup	1	250	1190
Beans, Dry, Most Varieties, Not Canned:				
▲Lentils, Boiled	1 cup	1	230	0
Lima, Boiled:				
▲Fresh	1 cup	1	210	30
▲Baby, Frozen	1 cup	1	190	50
▲Fordhook, Frozen	1 cup	1	170	90
▲Split Peas, Boiled	1 cup	1	230	0
▲White Beans, Boiled	1 cup	1	250	10
Beans, Other Products:				
▲ Falafel	3 patties	9	170	150
▲ Hummus, Homemade	1/2 cup	10	210	30
Peanuts:				
▲ Dry Roasted, Salted	1/4 cup	18	210	300
▲ Oil Roasted, Salted	1/4 cup	18	210	160
▲ Dry Or Oil Roasted, Unsalted	1/4 cup	18	210	0
▲ Reduced Fat, Honey Roasted, PLANTERS®	1/3 cup	7	130	150
Peanut Butter, Added Salt:				
▲ Chunk Style	2 tablespoons	16	190	160
▲ Smooth	2 tablespoons	16	190	150
▲ Reduced Fat, Chunky, SKIPPY®	2 tablespoons	12	190	17
Soybeans And Products:				
▲Boiled, Plain	1/2 cup	8	150	0
▲Roasted, Dry	1/4 cup	9	190	0
▲Miso	1/2 cup	8	280	5030
▲Natto	1/2 cup	10	190	10
▲Soy Milk (Use as Milk Substitute)	1 cup	5	80	30
▲Tempeh	1/2 cup	6	170	10
Tofu (Soybean Curd):				
▲▲ Raw, Firm	1/2 cup	11	180	20
▲Raw, Regular	1/2 cup	6	90	10
Nuts And Seeds:				
Almonds, Dry, Roasted:				
▲ Unsalted	1 oz.	15	170	0
▲ Salted	1 oz.	15	170	130
▲ Brazilnuts, Medium, Dried, Unsalted	2 oz. (16)	38	370	0

Protein Foods

FOOD	SERVING SIZE	FAT GMS	CALS	NA MGS
Nuts And Seeds (Continued):				
Cashews, Medium, Oil Roasted:				
▲ Unsalted	1 oz. (18)	14	160	10
▲ Salted	1 oz. (18)	15	170	110
Coconut, Dried, Sweetened, Flaked, Packaged	1/4 cup	6	90	50
Macadamia Nuts, Dried	1 oz.	21	200	0
Mixed Nuts With Peanuts:				
▲ Dry Roasted, Salted	1 oz.	15	170	190
▲ Oil Roasted, Salted	1 oz.	16	180	180
Peanuts (See Under Legumes):				
Pecan Halves, Large, Dried, Unsalted	1 oz. (31)	19	190	0
Pistachios, Dried	1 oz. (47)	14	160	0
Pumpkin & Squash Seeds:				
▲ Roasted, Unsalted	1 oz.	12	150	10
▲ Roasted, Salted	1 oz.	12	150	160
▲ Sesame Butter (Tahini)	2 tablespoons	16	180	30
Sesame Seeds, Unsalted	1 tablespoon	4	50	0
▲Soybean Nuts, Roasted	1/4 cup	11	200	70
▲ Sunflower Seeds, Dry Roasted, Unsalted	1 oz.	14	170	0
▲ Walnuts, Black, Dried	1 oz.	16	170	0
Walnuts, English, Dried	1 oz.	18	180	0
Organ Meats:				
▲Heart, Beef, Simmered	3 oz.	5	150	50
▲Kidney, Beef, Simmered	3 oz.	3	120	120
Liver:				
▲Beef, Fried	3 oz.	7	190	90
▲Chicken, Simmered	3 oz.	5	130	40
▲Chitterlings, Simmered	3 oz.	25	260	30
Pork, Fresh, Uncured:				
Chops:				
Loin Chops, Fried:				
▲Lean & Fat	3 oz.	14	240	70
▲Lean Only	3 oz.	9	200	70
Rib Chops, Broiled:				
▲Lean & Fat	3 oz.	13	220	50
▲Lean Only	3 oz.	8	190	60
Ribs, Lean & Fat:				
▲Back Ribs, Roasted	3 oz.	25	320	90
▲Country Style, Braised	3 oz.	18	250	50
▲Spareribs, Braised	3 oz.	26	340	80
Shoulder, Roasted:				
▲Lean & Fat	3 oz.	18	250	60
▲Lean Only	3 oz.	11	190	70
▲Tenderloin, Lean Only, Roasted	3 oz.	4	140	50
Pork Products, Cured:				
Bacon, Cooked	3 slices	9	110	300
▲Canadian Bacon, Grilled	2 oz.	5	100	870
Ham:				
▲Boiled, OSCAR MAYER®	2.25 oz.	3	60	820
▲Center Slice, Lean & Fat	3 oz.	11	170	1180
▲5% Fat	3 oz.	5	120	1020
▲11% Fat	3 oz.	8	150	1280
▲Lower NA, OSCAR MAYER®	2.5 oz.	3	70	520
Salt Pork, Raw	1 oz.	23	210	400

Protein Foods

FOOD	SERVING SIZE	FAT GMS	CALS	NA MGS
Poultry:				
Chicken, Broilers/Fryers,				
No Salt added:				
Breast, Meat & Skin:				
▲Fried, With Flour	1/2 breast	9	220	80
▲Roasted	1/2 breast	8	190	70
▲Breast, Meat Only,				
Roasted	1/2 breast	3	140	60
Drumstick, Meat & Skin:				
▲Fried, With Flour	1 drumstick	7	120	40
▲Roasted	1 drumstick	6	110	50
▲Drumstick, Meat Only,				
Roasted	1 drumstick	3	80	40
Thigh, Meat & Skin:				
▲Fried, With Flour	1 thigh	9	160	60
▲Roasted	1 thigh	10	150	50
▲Thigh, Meat Only,				
Roasted	1 thigh	6	110	50
▲Wing, Meat & Skin,				
Fried, With Flour	1 wing	7	100	30
▲Wing, Meat Only,				
Roasted	1 wing	2	40	20
▲Duck, Domestic, Meat				
Only, Roasted	1/2 duck (approx. 8 oz.)	25	450	140
▲Goose, Domestic, Meat				
Only, Roasted	4 oz.	14	270	90
Turkey:				
▲Ground, Cooked	2 oz.	8	130	50
Roasted, With Skin:				
▲Light Meat	2 oz.	5	110	40
▲Dark Meat	2 oz.	7	120	40
▲Oven Roasted, OSCAR MEYER®	2 oz.	1	50	620
Roasted, Without Skin:				
▲Light Meat	2 oz.	2	90	40
▲Dark Meat	2 oz.	4	100	40
Sausages And Luncheon Meats:				
HORMEL® Canned Meat Products:				
Chunk Meats:				
▲Chunk Chicken Breast	2 oz.	2	60	100
▲Chunk Chicken	2 oz.	3	70	200
▲ Chunk Ham	2 oz.	6	90	600
▲ Chunk Turkey	2 oz.	3	70	340
▲Chunk White Turkey	2 oz.	1	60	320
▲ Chunk Turkey Ham	2 oz.	4	70	600
▲Corned Beef	2 oz.	7	120	490
▲ Pickled Pigs Feet	2 oz.	6	80	530
▲ Roast Beef With Gravy	2 oz.	2	60	280
▲ Sliced Dried Beef	10 slices (1 oz.)	2	50	1240
SPAM®:				
▲ Luncheon Meat	2 oz.	16	170	750
▲ Lite	2 oz.	8	110	560
▲ Less Salt	2 oz.	16	170	560
Spreads:				
▲ Deviled Ham	4 tablespoons	12	150	430
▲ SPAM®	4 tablespoons	11	130	580
▲ Liverwurst	4 tablespoons	10	130	650

Protein Foods

FOOD	SERVING SIZE	FAT GMS	CALS	NA MGS
Sausages And Luncheon Meats (Continued):				
HORMEL® Canned Meat Products (Continued):				
▲ Vienna Sausage	2 oz.	13	140	420
▲ Vienna Chicken Sausage	2 oz.	10	110	420
HORMEL® Deli Meats:				
▲ Deli Cooked Ham	2 oz.	2	60	690
▲ Pepperoni, Sliced	15 slices (1 oz.)	13	140	470
▲ Roast Beef, Top Round	2 oz.	1	50	580
HORMEL® Franks:				
▲ Cocktail Wieners	5 wieners	14	160	550
▲ Corn Dogs	2.75 oz.	11	220	520
▲ LIGHT & LEAN® 97	1 frank	1	50	490
▲ Meat Franks	1 (10/1#)	13	140	430
HORMEL® Ham:				
▲CUREMASTER® Ham	3 oz.	3	80	940
▲LIGHT & LEAN® Ham	3 oz.	3	90	950
▲PRIMISSIMO®	2 oz.	9	140	1080
LOUIS RICH®:				
Chicken Breast:				
▲ Oven Roasted	2 slices (2 oz.)	5	80	700
▲ Oven Roasted, DELI-THIN®	4 slices (2 oz.)	2	60	620
▲CARVING BOARD™	3 slices (2.4 oz.)	1	60	800
Turkey:				
▲ Bacon	4 slices (2 oz.)	10	120	760
▲ Breast, Barbecued	2 oz.	1	60	630
▲ Frank, Turkey & Chicken	1	6	80	480
▲ Ground	2 oz.	6	100	70
▲ Ham, Chopped	2 slices (2 oz.)	5	80	580
▲ Hickory Smoked, DELI-THIN®	4 slices (2 oz.)	1	50	490
▲ Polska Kielbasa	2 oz.	5	80	500
▲ Sausage Links	2 links	6	90	470
▲ Smoked Sausage	2 oz.	5	80	500
LOUIS RICH® Fat Free Products, Turkey Breast:				
▲ DELI-THIN®	4 slices (2 oz.)	0	40	610
▲ Hickory Smoked	2 slices (2 oz.)	0	50	600
MR. TURKEY®, Turkey Products:				
▲ Bologna	2 slices	10	140	740
▲ Cotto Salami	2 slices	7	100	480
▲ Breast, Roasted	2 slices	2	60	540
▲Ground (91% fat free)	3.5 oz.	10	170	90
▲ Ham	2 slices	3	70	740
▲ Sausage, Hot Smoked, Polish Kielbasa	2 oz.	5	90	500
▲ Pastrami	2 slices	2	60	580
OSCAR MAYER®:				
▲ Bologna, Beef	2 slices (2 oz.)	16	180	600
▲ Bologna, Beef Light	2 slices (2 oz.)	8	120	620
▲ Bologna, Pork, Chicken & Beef	2 slices (2 oz.)	16	180	540
▲ Braunschweiger	2 oz.	18	200	640
▲ Ham, Honey, HEALTHY FAVORITES™	4 slices (2 oz.)	2	50	630
▲ Roast Beef, DELI-THIN®	4 slices (2 oz.)	2	60	530
▲ Salami, Hard, DELI-THIN®	4 slices (1 oz.)	11	130	620

Protein Foods

FOOD	SERVING SIZE	FAT GMS	CALS	NA MGS
OSCAR MAYER® (Continued):				
▲ Summer Sausage, Thuringer Cervelat	2 slices (2 oz.)	13	140	650
▲ Turkey Breast Roasted, DELI-THIN®	4 slices (1 oz.)	1	50	580
Wieners:				
▲ Original	1	22	240	690
▲ Original Beef Franks	1	22	240	700
▲ BUN-LENGTH™	1	17	190	570
OSCAR MAYER® FREE® Fat Free Products:				
▲ Bologna, Turkey, Beef, Pork	2 slices (2 oz.)	0	40	480
▲ Chicken Breast, Oven Roasted	4 slices (2 oz.)	0	50	650
▲ Hot Dogs, Turkey & Beef	1	0	40	460
▲ Turkey Breast, Oven Roasted	4 slices (2 oz.)	0	40	610
▲ Turkey Breast, Smoked	4 slices (2 oz.)	0	40	550
Sausage:				
▲Italian, Pork	1 link (2.5 oz.)	17	220	620
▲▲▲▲Polish	1 (8 oz.)	65	740	1990
▲ Pork	1 oz. or 2 links	8	100	350
▲ Pork & Beef	1 oz. or 2 links	9	100	210
▲Veal, Roasted	3 oz.	10	200	70

FATS, OILS AND SALAD DRESSINGS

Butter:				
Salted	1 teaspoon	4	40	40
Unsalted	1 teaspoon	4	40	0
Lard	1 tablespoon	13	120	0
Margarine:				
Salted	1 teaspoon	4	30	40
Unsalted	1 teaspoon	4	30	0
CHIFFON® Soft	1 tablespoon	11	100	110
CHIFFON® Whipped	1 tablespoon	7	70	70
PARKAY® Soft Diet	1 tablespoon	6	50	110
PARKAY® Squeeze	1 tablespoon	9	80	120
Oil, Vegetable	1 tablespoon	14	120	0
Salad Dressing, Commercial:				
Blue Cheese	1 tablespoon	8	80	?-
French:				
Low Calorie	1 tablespoon	1	20	130
Regular	1 tablespoon	6	70	210
Italian:				
Low Calorie	1 tablespoon	2	20	120
Regular	1 tablespoon	7	70	120
Russian:				
Low Calorie	1 tablespoon	1	20	140
Regular	1 tablespoon	8	80	130
Thousand Island:				
Low Calorie	1 tablespoon	2	20	150
Regular	1 tablespoon	6	60	110
Salad Dressing, HIDDEN VALLEY®:				
Blue Cheese, Regular	2 tablespoons	17	160	260
Blue Cheese, Lowfat	2 tablespoons	0	20	270
Creamy Parmesan, Regular	2 tablespoons	15	140	260

Protein Foods and Fats and Oils

FOOD	SERVING SIZE	FAT GMS	CALS	NA MGS
Salad Dressing, HIDDEN VALLEY® (Continued):				
Creamy Parmesan, Lowfat	2 tablespoons	0	30	250
Italian Parmesan, Lowfat	2 tablespoons	0	20	240
Original Ranch, Regular	2 tablespoons	14	140	260
Original Ranch, Lowfat	2 tablespoons	3	40	270
Original Ranch, Reduced Calorie	2 tablespoons	7	80	270
Salad Dressing, KRAFT®, Mayonnaise And Mayonnaise Type Dressing:				
KRAFT FREE® Fat Free	1 tablespoon	0	10	110
KRAFT LIGHT®	1 tablespoon	5	50	110
KRAFT® Real Mayonnaise	1 tablespoon	11	100	80
MIRACLE WHIP® FREE® Nonfat	1 tablespoon	0	20	120
MIRACLE WHIP® LIGHT®	1 tablespoon	3	40	120
MIRACLE WHIP® Regular	1 tablespoon	7	70	90
KRAFT FREE® Fat Free Dressing:				
Blue Cheese Flavor	2 tablespoons	0	50	340
French Style	2 tablespoons	0	50	300
Italian	2 tablespoons	0	10	290
Ranch	2 tablespoons	0	50	310
KRAFT® DELICIOUSLY RIGHT® Reduced Calorie Dressing:				
CATALINA® French	2 tablespoons	4	80	400
Creamy Italian	2 tablespoons	5	50	250
Cucumber French	2 tablespoons	5	60	450
KRAFT® Regular Dressing:				
Buttermilk Ranch	2 tablespoons	16	150	230
Caesar	2 tablespoons	13	130	370
Catalina® French	2 tablespoons	11	140	390
Coleslaw	2 tablespoons	12	150	420
Creamy Italian	2 tablespoons	11	110	230
Sandwich Spread, Commercial	1 tablespoon	5	60	?-
Shortening, Vegetable Oil, Hydrogenated	1 tablespoon	13	110	?-

DESSERTS AND SWEETS

FOOD	SERVING SIZE	FAT GMS	CALS	NA MGS
Cakes Baked From Mixes:				
Boston Cream Pie	1/8 cake	6	270	390
Chocolate Pudding	1/6 cake	5	230	250
Gingerbread, From Mix	1/9 cake	4	170	190
Yellow, Chocolate Icing	1/12 cake	11	260	350
Cake Icing From Mix Or Ready To Spread	Amount for 1/12 cake	7	150	70
DUNCAN HINES®, No Icing:				
Moist Deluxe:				
Butter Recipe Golden	1/10 cake	16	320	190
Spice	1/12 cake	11	250	270
White	1/12 cake	10	240	220
Yellow Delights	1/10 cake	5	220	320
PILLSBURY PLUS®, No Icing:				
Angel Food Cake	1/10 cake	0	150	360
Carrot Cake	1/12 cake	12	260	300
Chocolate Cake	1/12 cake	12	260	330
Chocolate Chip Cake	1/12 cake	10	240	280
Double Hot Fudge Bundt	1/16 cake	16	280	220
LOVIN' LITES® Devil's Food	1/10 cake	5	230	420

Fats and Oils and Desserts and Sweets

FOOD	SERVING SIZE	FAT GMS	CALS	NA MGS
Candy:				
Butterscotch	5 pieces (1 oz.)	1	120	20
Caramels, Plain	4 pieces (1 oz.)	2	120	80
Caramels, Chocolate	5 pieces (1 oz.)	1	110	?-
Chocolate Covered Peanuts	30 pieces (1 oz.)	10	150	10
Chocolate Chips, Semi-Sweet	1 cup	50	800	20
Fudge, With Nuts	1 oz.	3	110	30
Gum Drops	10 small (1 oz.)	0	140	20
Hard Candy	1 oz.	0	110	10
Jelly Beans	10 large (1 oz.)	0	100	10
Marshmallow, Plain	3 large	0	70	10
Milk Chocolate, With Peanuts	7 pieces (1 oz.)	9	150	10
M&M's®, Plain	15 pieces	2	50	10
M&M's®, With Peanuts	15 pieces	8	150	30
Peanut Brittle	1 oz.	5	130	130
REECE'S® Peanut Butter Cups	6 small cups (1.5 oz.)	13	200	120
YORK® Peppermint Patty	1 small	1	40	0
Cookies:				
Brownie With Nuts, Homemade	1 (3" x 1" x 1")	6	100	50
Brownie With Nuts, Homemade, Chocolate Frosting	1 (1.5" x 2" x 1")	5	100	50
Chocolate, Commercial	2 cookies (.75 oz.)	4	100	80
Chocolate Chip, Homemade	2 cookies (.75 oz.)	5	90	40
Chocolate Coated Graham Cracker	2 squares (1 oz.)	6	120	110
Ginger Snaps, SUNSHINE®	5 cookies	3	100	120
Graham Cracker, Cinnamon, SUNSHINE®	2 squares	3	70	100
Oatmeal With Raisins, Commercial	2 (1 oz.)	4	120	40
Vanilla Wafers	5 cookies	3	90	50
HYDROX®:				
Regular	3 cookies	7	150	130
Reduced Fat	3 cookies	4	130	140
KEEBLER®:				
CHIPS DELUXE® Chocolate Chip:				
Regular	1 cookie (.5 oz.)	5	80	60
25% Reduced Fat	1 cookie (.5 oz.)	3	70	70
Fudge Shoppe® Deluxe Grahams, Fudge Covered	3 cookies (1 oz.)	7	140	110
PECAN SANDIES® Rich Shortbread:				
Regular	1 cookie (.5 oz.)	5	80	80
25% Reduced Fat	1 cookie (.5 oz.)	3	70	50
ELFINS DELIGHTS®:				
50% Reduced Fat Chocolate Sandwich	2 cookies	3	110	100
Fat Free Devil's Food	1 cookie	0	70	80
Golden Vanilla Wafers	8 cookies	7	150	120
Golden Vanilla Wafers, 30% Reduced Fat	8 cookies	4	130	140
KEEBLER GRAHAM SELECTS®:				
Old Fashioned	8 crackers	6	150	140
LOW FAT CINNAMON CRISP®	8 crackers	2	110	190
Low Fat Honey Graham	9 crackers	2	120	210

Desserts and Sweets

FOOD	SERVING SIZE	FAT GMS	CALS	NA MGS
NABISCO®:				
Arrowroot Biscuit, National®	2 cookies	1	40	30
CHIPS AHOY!® Chocolate Cookies:				
Regular	3 cookies	8	170	130
Reduced Fat	3 cookies	6	150	150
FIG NEWTONS®:				
Regular	2 cookies	3	110	120
Fat Free	2 cookies	0	100	120
Grahams:				
Regular	8 crackers	3	120	180
HONEY MAID®:				
Cinnamon	10 crackers	3	140	210
Honey	8 crackers	3	120	180
OREO® Chocolate Sandwich:				
Regular	3 cookies	7	160	220
Reduced Fat	3 cookies	5	140	190
SNACKWELL'S® Reduced Fat Sandwich:				
Chocolate/Chocolate Creme	2 cookies	3	100	190
Vanilla/Vanilla Creme	2 cookies	3	110	100
SNACKWELL'S® Fat Free:				
Devil's Food Cookie Cakes	1 cookie	0	50	30
Double Fudge Cookie Cakes	1 cookie	0	50	70
Desserts, Frozen:				
Fruit & Juice Bars	1 bar (3 oz.)	0	80	0
Gelatin Pops	1 pop	0	30	20
Ice Cream, 10% Fat	1/2 cup	7	130	60
Ice Milk, Vanilla:				
Hardened	1/2 cup	3	90	60
Soft Serve	1/2 cup	2	110	60
Ice Pops	1 bar (2 oz.)	0	40	0
Pudding Pop, Chocolate	1 pop	2	70	80
Sherbet, Orange	1/2 cup	2	130	40
Yogurt, Soft Serve:				
Chocolate	1/2 cup	4	120	70
Vanilla	1/2 cup	4	110	60
Dessert, Gelatin:				
Plain	1/2 cup	0	80	60
Plain, With Sugar Substitute	1/2 cup	0	10	60
With Fruit	1/2 cup	0	70	30
Desserts, Homemade:				
Apple Crisp	1/2 cup	5	230	260
Bread Pudding	1/2 cup	7	210	290
Cheesecake	1 piece (3 oz.)	16	260	190
Egg Custard	1/2 cup	7	150	110
Dessert Toppings:				
Butterscotch Or Caramel	2 tablespoons	0	100	140
Chocolate Syrup, Thin Type	2 tablespoons	0	80	40
Chocolate Syrup, Fudge Type	1 tablespoon	3	70	30
Strawberry	2 tablespoons	0	110	10
Whipped Topping:				
Cream, Whipped, Canned, Pressurized	2 tablespoons	1	20	10
From Mix, DREAM WHIP®	2 tablespoons	1	20	10
From Mix, NUTRASWEET®, D-ZERTA®	2 tablespoons	1	10	10
Frozen, COOL WHIP®, Lite Or Extra Creamy Or Non-Dairy	2 tablespoons	2	30	10

Desserts and Sweets

FOOD	SERVING SIZE	FAT GMS	CALS	NA MGS
Desserts, Ready-To-Eat:				
ENTENMANN'S® Baked Goods:				
Apple Strudel	1/4 strudel	14	310	230
Carrot Cake	1/8 cake	16	290	240
Homestyle Apple Pie	1/6 pie	14	300	300
Marshmallow Iced Devil's Food Cake	1/6 cake	18	350	290
ENTENMANN'S® Fat Free Cholesterol Free Sweet Baked Goods:				
Apple Beehive Pie	1/5 pie	0	270	330
Apple Buns	1 bun	0	150	140
Carrot Cake	1/8 cake	0	170	230
Chocolate Brownie	2 brownies	0	80	90
Chocolate Crunch Cake	1/8 cake	0	130	170
Oatmeal Raisin Cookies	2 cookies	0	80	120
Doughnut, Plain:				
Cake Type	1 (1 oz.)	6	110	140
Glazed, HOSTESS®	1 (2 oz.)	12	230	200
Powdered Sugar, HOSTESS®	1 (1 oz.)	5	110	140
Ice Cream Cone, No Ice Cream	1 cone	0	50	30
Pies, PET RITZ®, Frozen:				
Crust, Regular	1/8 (9" crust)	5	80	60
Crust, Graham Cracker	1/8	6	110	120
Chocolate Cream Pie	1/4 pie	13	290	270
Peanut Butter Chocolate	1/4 pie	15	300	180
Pumpkin Cream	1/4 pie	13	270	250
Pies, Homemade (9 Inch):				
Apple	1/8 pie	12	280	180
Butterscotch	1/8 pie	13	300	240
Cherry	1/8 pie	13	310	360
Custard	1/8 pie	13	250	330
Lemon Meringue	1/6 pie	13	350	260
Pecan	1/8 pie	24	430	230
Pumpkin	1/8 pie	13	240	240
Puddings:				
Chocolate, Made From Mix With 2% Milk:				
Instant	1/2 cup	3	150	420
Noninstant	1/2 cup	3	150	150
Vanilla, Made From Mix With 2% Milk:				
Instant	1/2 cup	2	150	410
Noninstant	1/2 cup	2	140	220
Sugar:				
Brown, Packed	1/4 cup	0	210	20
White, Granulated	1/4 cup	0	190	0
White, Granulated	1 tablespoon	0	50	0
Sweet Roll, Commercial:				
Danish Pastry, Plain	1 (1.5 oz.)	9	160	160
Cinnamon Raisin	1 (2.25 oz.)	2	180	250
Syrup:				
Corn, Dark	1 tablespoon	0	60	30
Corn, Light	1 tablespoon	0	60	20
Cane Maple Blend	1 tablespoon	0	60	20
Molasses	1 tablespoon	0	50	10
Pancake, Reduced Calorie	2 tablespoons	0	50	60
Toppings, Bread:				
Apple Butter	1 tablespoon	0	30	0
Honey	1 tablespoon	0	60	0
Jams, Jellies, & Preserves	1 tablespoon	0	50	10

Desserts and Sweets

FOOD	SERVING SIZE	FAT GMS	CALS	NA MGS
MISCELLANEOUS				
Baking Powder:				
Calumet	1 teaspoon	0	0	430
Cream Of Tartar	1 teaspoon	0	0	230
Beverages:				
Alcoholic:				
Beer, Regular	12 oz.	0	150	20
Beer, Light	12 oz.	0	100	10
Bloody Mary Cocktail	5 oz.	0	120	330
Daiquiri	2 oz.	0	110	0
Martini, No Olives	2.5 oz.	0	160	0
Pina Colada	4.5 oz.	3	260	10
Gin & Whiskey	1.5 oz.	0	110	0
Rum & Vodka	1.5 oz.	0	100	0
Coffee Liqueur	1.5 oz.	0	170	0
Creme De Menthe	1.5 oz.	0	190	0
Wine:				
Table, All	3.5 oz.	0	70	10
Dessert, All	2 oz.	0	90	10
Cooler	12 oz.	0	220	10
Carbonated:				
Club Soda	12 oz.	0	0	80
Cream Soda	12 oz.	0	190	40
Cola Type	12 oz.	0	150	10
Diet Soda, Cola, With Aspartame	12 oz.	0	0	20
Ginger Ale	12 oz.	0	120	30
Grape	12 oz.	0	160	60
Lemon-Lime	12 oz.	0	150	40
Mineral Water	12 oz.	0	0	?-
Orange	12 oz.	0	180	50
Pepper-Type	12 oz.	0	150	40
Root Beer	12 oz.	0	150	50
Tonic Or Quinine	12 oz.	0	130	20
Cocoa Mix Powder	1 packet	3	120	210
Coffee:				
Brewed	6 oz.	0	0	0
Brewed	12 oz.	0	0	10
Flavors From Instant:				
Cappucino	2 rounded tsp.	2	60	100
French	2 rounded tsp.	3	60	?-
Plain Powder	Any amount	0	0	0
Eggnog	1 cup	19	340	140
Instant Breakfast, Vanilla, No Sugar Added, CARNATION®	1 envelope & 1 c. 2% milk	5	190	240
Lemonade Flavor Powder	2 tablespoons	0	110	10
Malted Milk Powder, Natural	3 rounded tsp.	2	90	100
Orange Flavor Drink Powder	3 rounded tsp.	0	90	0
Postum®	1 teaspoon	0	10	0
Tea:				
Brewed	12 oz.	0	0	10
Plain Powder	1 teaspoon	0	0	0
Plain Powder	12 teaspoons	0	0	10
Lemon Flavor Powder With Sugar	3 rounded tsp.	0	90	?-
Catsup, Tomato	1 tablespoon	0	20	180
Chocolate, Baking Or Bitter	1 square (1 oz.)	16	150	0

Miscellaneous

FOOD	SERVING SIZE	FAT GMS	CALS	NA MGS
Cocoa, Dry Powder, Not Dutch Process	1 tablespoon	0	10	0
Gravy, Dehydrated, Au Jus	1 packet	3	80	2390
Horseradish	1 tablespoon	0	10	10
Mustard, Prepared, Yellow	1 teaspoon	0	0	60
Nuts And Seeds (See Protein Foods)				
Olives, Pitted:				
Green	10 large	5	50	930
Ripe	10 large	5	50	380
Pickles:				
Dill	1 large (3.75" long)	0	10	830
Dill	2 slices	0	0	150
Sweet Gherkin	1 large (3" long)	0	40	330
Sweet Relish	1 tablespoon	0	20	120
Salt:				
Garlic	1 teaspoon	0	0	1300
Lite	1 teaspoon	0	0	1100
Table	1 teaspoon	0	0	2300
Salt Substitute	1 teaspoon	0	0	0
Sauces:				
HEALTHY CHOICE®:				
Barbecue:				
Original	2 tablespoons	0	20	230
Hot & Spicy	2 tablespoons	0	20	230
Pasta Sauces:				
Traditional	1/2 cup	1	50	390
Garlic & Herbs	1/2 cup	1	50	390
Extra Chunky Italian	1/2 cup	0	40	380
HUNT'S® Sauces:				
CHICKEN SENSATIONS®:				
Italian Garlic	1 tablespoon	3	30	330
Lemon Herb	1 tablespoon	3	30	380
HUNT'S® Spaghetti Sauce:				
Original Traditional	1/2 cup	2	70	620
Home Style & Mushrooms	1/2 cup	3	60	590
Chunky Marinara	1/2 cup	2	60	530
KRAFT®:				
Barbecue:				
Extra Rich, Original	2 tablespoons	0	50	360
Mesquite Smoke	2 tablespoons	0	50	440
Miscellaneous KRAFT® Sauces:				
Cream Style Horseradish	2 teaspoons	0	10	100
Nonfat Tartar Sauce	2 tablespoons	0	30	210
SAUCEWORKS® Tartar Sauce	2 tablespoons	10	100	180
PROGRESSO® Pasta Sauces:				
Alfredo, Authentic	1/2 cup	27	310	670
Marinara, Authentic	1/2 cup	5	100	440
White Clam, Authentic	1/2 cup	7	90	470
Miscellaneous Other Sauces:				
Soy Sauce, KIKKOMAN®	2 tablespoons	0	20	1540
Soy Sauce, KIKKOMAN®, Lite	2 tablespoons	0	20	960
Tartar	1 tablespoon	8	70	190
Taco, Mild ROSARITA®	3 tablespoons	0	20	310
Teriyaki	1 tablespoon	0	20	690
Worcestershire	1 tablespoon	0	10	230

Miscellaneous

FOOD	SERVING SIZE	FAT GMS	CALS	NA MGS
Snack Foods:				
Banana Chips	1 oz.	10	150	0
Beef Jerky	1 oz.	4	100	820
Chex Party Mix, RALSTON®:				
Bold & Zesty	1/2 cup	7	160	390
Golden Cheddar Cheese	2/3 cup	5	140	250
Traditional Flavor	2/3 cup	4	130	280
CHEEZ-IT® Party Mix	1/2 cup	5	140	270
Corn Chips, Plain	1 oz.	7	140	150
Corn Nuts, Plain	1 oz.	4	120	160
DORITO THINS®, Original	1 oz. (9 chips)	7	140	140
TOSTITOS®, Baked, Lowfat	1 oz. (13 chips)	1	110	140
Tortilla Chips, Baked Not Fried, GUILTLESS GOURMET®:				
Chili & Lime	1 oz. (20 chips)	1	110	200
Original Style	1 oz. (20 chips)	1	110	160
Original Style, No Salt	1 oz. (20 chips)	1	110	30
Dips, GUILTLESS GOURMET®:				
BBQ Pinto Bean, Spicy	2 tablespoons	0	40	110
Black Bean, Spicy	2 tablespoons	0	30	100
Nacho, Spicy	2 tablespoons	0	30	150
Dips, KRAFT®:				
Avocado	2 tablespoons	4	60	240
Clam	2 tablespoons	4	60	250
Blue Cheese, Premium	2 tablespoons	4	50	200
French Onion	2 tablespoons	4	60	230
Jalapeno Bean	2 tablespoons	4	60	260
Ranch	2 tablespoons	4	60	210
Dips, OLD EL PASO®:				
Black Bean	2 tablespoons	0	20	150
Cheese 'n Salsa, Mild	2 tablespoons	3	40	300
Jalapeno	2 tablespoons	1	30	130
Popcorn, Popped:				
Air-Popped, Unsalted	3 cups	1	90	0
Caramel Coated & Peanuts	2/3 cup	2	110	80
Cheese Flavored	3 cups	11	170	290
Popcorn, Popped:				
With Oil & Salt	3 cups	9	170	290
Pork Rinds	1 oz.	9	150	520
Potato Chips:				
Chips	1 oz.	10	150	170
Chips, Light	1 oz.	6	130	140
FRITO LAY®:				
Reduced Fat, Baked	1 oz. (11 chips)	2	110	210
RUFFLES®, Regular	1 oz. (17 chips)	10	160	180
RUFFLES®, Reduced Fat	1 oz. (16 chips)	7	140	130
PRINGLES® Crisps:				
Cheez-ums	1 oz. (14 chips)	10	150	190
Original	1 oz. (14 chips)	11	160	170
Ranch	1 oz. (14 chips)	10	150	130
PRINGLES RIGHT CRISPS®:				
Original	1 oz (16 chips)	7	140	140
Ranch or Sour Cream & Onion	1 oz. (16 chips)	7	140	120
PRINGLES RIPPLES®	1 oz. (10 chips)	11	160	150
Potato Sticks	1/2 cup	6	90	50

Miscellaneous

FOOD	SERVING SIZE	FAT GMS	CALS	NA MGS
Pretzels:				
Hard, Plain	2 oz.	2	230	1030
MISTER SALTY®:				
Dutch Pretzels	1 oz. (2 pretzels)	1	120	580
Pretzel Sticks, Fat Free	1 oz. (47 pretzels)	0	110	370
Pretzel Twists, Fat Free	1 oz. (9 pretzels)	0	110	380
Sesame Sticks	1 oz.	10	150	420
Soups:				
Commercial, Canned:				
Cream Type Condensed:				
Cheese	1 can (11 oz.)	25	380	2330
Chicken	1 can (11 oz.)	18	280	2400
Mushroom	1 can (11 oz.)	23	310	2470
Pea, Green	1 can (11 oz.)	7	400	2400
Potato	1 can (11 oz.)	6	180	2430
Tomato	1 can (11 oz.)	5	210	2120
Prepared With Whole Milk:				
Cheese	1 cup	15	230	1020
Chicken	1 cup	11	190	1050
Mushroom	1 cup	14	200	1080
Pea, Green	1 cup	7	250	1050
Potato	1 cup	6	150	1060
Tomato	1 cup	6	160	930
Prepared With Water:				
Chicken Noodle	1 cup	2	80	1110
Vegetable/Beef	1 cup	2	80	960
Dehydrated Form, Broth Or Bouillon:				
Beef	1 cube	0	5	860
Beef	1 packet	1	10	1020
Chicken	1 cube	0	10	1150
Onion Mix	1 packet	2	120	3490
HEALTHY CHOICE®:				
Clam Chowder	1 cup	1	120	480
Country Vegetable	1 cup	1	100	430
Cream Of Mushroom	1 cup	1	80	450
Split Pea & Ham	1 cup	2	160	400
Vegetable Beef	1 cup	1	130	420
HEALTH VALLEY®, Fat Free:				
Black Bean & Vegetable	1 cup	0	110	280
5-Bean Vegetable	1 cup	0	140	250
Lentil & Carrots	1 cup	0	90	220
Pasta Romano	1 cup	0	140	250
Split Pea & Carrots	1 cup	0	110	230
PROGRESSO®:				
Beans & Ham	1 cup	2	160	870
Beef Vegetable & Rotini	1 cup	4	120	830
Clam & Rotini Chowder	1 cup	9	200	800
Corn Chowder	1 cup	10	180	780
Green Split Pea	1 cup	3	170	870
HEALTHY CLASSICS®:				
Beef Vegetable	1 cup	2	150	410
N.E. Clam Chowder	1 cup	2	120	530
Split Pea	1 cup	3	180	420
Hearty Minestrone/Shells	1 cup	2	120	700
Hearty Vegetable/Rotini	1 cup	1	110	720
Lentil	1 can (10.5 oz.)	3	170	930
Vinegar, Cider	1 cup	0	30	0

Miscellaneous

FOOD	SERVING SIZE	FAT GMS	CALS	NA MGS
FROZEN, CANNED, AND BOXED ENTREES AND MEALS:				
Boxed Entrees, Prepared:				
BETTY CROCKER® Helper Meals, Mix Only:				
Hamburger Helper:				
Beef Taco	1/5 package	2	160	870
Nacho Cheese	1/5 package	3	160	870
Swedish Meatballs	1/5 package	7	170	750
Tuna Helper:				
Au Gratin	1/5 package	4	190	770
Tetrazzini	1/5 package	3	180	790
KRAFT®, Prepared:				
Cheddar Cheese Egg Noodle	1 cup	21	430	780
Original Macaroni & Cheese Dinner	1 cup	17	390	730
VELVEETA® Rotini & Cheese With Broccoli	1 cup	16	400	1240
KRAFT® Pasta Salads, Prepared:				
Classic Ranch With Bacon	3/4 cup	23	360	500
Garden Primavera	3/4 cup	12	280	730
Parmesan Peppercorn	3/4 cup	25	360	610
Light Italian Pasta	3/4 cup	2	190	660
Canned Entrees & Dinners:				
DINTY MOORE® Canned Stews:				
Beef Stew	1 cup	14	230	950
Chicken Stew	1 cup	11	220	980
Meatball Stew	1 cup	16	260	1110
HORMEL®:				
Beans & Weiners	1 can (7.5 oz.)	13	290	1270
Chili With Beans	1 can (7.5 oz.)	11	250	1000
DINTY MOORE® Beef Stew	1 can (7.5 oz.)	10	190	870
MARY KITCHEN® Corned Beef Hash	1 can (7.5 oz.)	22	350	850
Turkey Chili With Beans	1 cup	3	220	1280
Tamales, Beef	3 tamales	21	280	1010
Tamales, Chicken	3 tamales	10	210	1040
HUNT'S® Homestyle Separates:				
Chili Fixings	1/2 cup	1	80	860
Noodles & Beef	1 cup	4	150	1240
Noodles & Chicken	1 cup	6	180	1280
Rigatoni & Italian Garden Sauce	1 cup	5	170	830
LA CHOY® Bi-Pack Dinners:				
Chicken Chow Mein	1 cup	4	110	1080
Beef Chow Mein	1 cup	2	110	760
Shrimp Chow Mein	1 cup	1	50	950
Pork Chow Mein	1 cup	2	80	1180
LA CHOY® Canned Entrees:				
Noodles & Vegetables	1 cup	1	130	1310
Noodles & Vegetables & Beef	1 cup	4	160	1330
Sweet & Sour Noodles & Chicken	1 cup	3	260	700
Chicken Chow Mein	1 cup	4	80	1350
Fried Rice	1 cup	1	240	1020

FOOD	SERVING SIZE	FAT GMS	CALS	NA MGS
Frozen Items:				
BANQUET® Pot Pies:				
Vegetable Pot Pie/Chicken	1 pie	18	350	950
Vegetable Pot Pie/Beef	1 pie	15	330	1000
Macaroni & Cheese Pot Pie	1 pie	3	200	600
BANQUET® Extra Helping Dinners:				
Fried Chicken	1 dinner	39	790	1820
Turkey	1 dinner	20	560	1910
Salisbury Steak	1 dinner	46	740	1860
Mexican Style	1 dinner	34	820	2060
BANQUET® Regular Frozen Dinners:				
BBQ Style Chicken	1 dinner	12	320	800
Fried Chicken	1 dinner	27	470	980
Meatloaf	1 dinner	17	280	1100
Chicken & Dumpling	1 dinner	8	260	780
Chimichanga Meal	1 dinner	23	470	1180
Beef Enchilada	1 dinner	12	320	1330
Oriental Style Chicken	1 dinner	9	260	610
CHICKEN BY GEORGE®:				
Lemon Herb	1 breast	3	120	800
Mesquite Barbecue	1 breast	2	120	800
Roasted	1 breast	3	110	500
CHUN KING® Egg Rolls:				
Pork & Shrimp	8 egg rolls	11	290	350
Shrimp	8 egg rolls	8	260	480
Chicken	8 egg rolls	9	270	350
CHUN KING® Meals:				
Chicken Chow Mein	1 meal	14	370	2010
Walnut Chicken	1 meal	19	460	1820
Beef Pepper Steak	1 meal	4	300	1670
Sweet & Sour Pork	1 meal	6	450	1180
GREEN GIANT®:				
Harvest Burgers®, Original	1 burger	4	140	380
Breakfast Patties	2 patties	4	100	280
Breakfast Links	3 links	5	110	340
HEALTHY CHOICE® Entrees:				
Beef Pepper Steak Oriental	1 meal	4	250	470
Country Glazed Chicken	1 meal	2	200	480
Fettuccine Alfredo	1 meal	5	250	480
Honey Mustard Chicken	1 meal	2	260	550
Lasagna Roma	1 meal	5	390	580
Spaghetti Bolognese	1 meal	3	260	470
HEALTHY CHOICE® Classics:				
Beef Broccoli Beijing	1 meal	3	330	500
Ginger Chicken Hunan	1 meal	3	350	430
Shrimp & Vegetables Maria	1 meal	3	270	540
Turkey Fettuccine Alla Crema	1 meal	4	350	370
HEALTHY CHOICE® Dinners:				
Beef & Peppers Cantonese	1 meal	5	270	560
Beef Tips With BBQ Sauce	1 meal	6	290	270
Chicken Cantonese	1 meal	1	210	360
Chicken Dijon	1 meal	4	280	410
Country Herb Chicken	1 meal	4	270	340
Shrimp Marinara	1 meal	1	220	220
Yankee Pot Roast	1 meal	5	280	460

Frozen, Canned, and Boxed Entrees and Meals

FOOD	SERVING SIZE	FAT GMS	CALS	NA MGS
Frozen Items (Continued):				
HORMEL® QUICK MEAL® Products:				
Hamburger	1 sandwich	15	350	360
Cheeseburger	1 sandwich	20	400	580
BBQ Beef	1 sandwich	16	360	560
Chicken	1 sandwich	12	340	480
Sausage Biscuit	1 sandwich	22	360	940
Beef Burrito	1 burrito	13	300	550
Cheese Burrito	1 burrito	6	250	640
Corn Dog	1 dog	11	220	520
LA CHOY® Egg Rolls:				
Pork, Restaurant Size	1 egg roll	6	170	390
Sweet & Sour, Restaurant Size	1 egg roll	4	180	300
Shrimp	3 egg rolls	5	170	420
MORTON®:				
Chicken Pot Pie	1 pie	18	320	1020
Beef Pot Pie	1 pie	17	310	1380
Fried Chicken Dinner	1 dinner	25	420	1000
Meatloaf Dinner	1 dinner	13	250	1110
Mexican Dinner	1 dinner	7	260	1000
OLD EL PASO® Frozen Items:				
Beef Chimichanga	1	20	370	470
Bean & Cheese Burrito	1	9	290	840
PATIO®:				
Mexican Dinner	1 dinner	15	440	1840
Beef Enchilada Dinner	1 dinner	8	320	1810
Fiesta Dinner	1 dinner	9	340	1760
Beef & Bean Burrito	1 burrito	7	280	860
Bean & Cheese Burrito	1 burrito	5	270	530
Chicken Burrito	1 burrito	4	260	740
RED BARON® Premium Pockets:				
Ham & Cheese	1 pocket	15	320	850
Chicken, Broccoli & Cheddar	1 pocket	13	290	540
STOUFFER'S® LEAN CUISINE®:				
Baked Chicken, Whipped Potatoes & Stuffing	1 entree	5	240	480
Beef Pot Roast & Whipped Potatoes	1 entree	7	210	570
Cafe Classics Bow Tie & Chicken	1 entree	6	270	550
Cafe Classics Calypso Chicken	1 entree	6	280	590
Chicken Chow Mein & Rice	1 entree	5	210	510
Fettucini Primavera	1 entree	8	260	580
Meatloaf & Whipped Potatoes	1 entree	7	250	570
Oriental Beef	1 entree	8	250	480
Roasted Turkey Breast & Stuffing & Cinnamon Apples	1 entree	4	290	530
Spaghetti With Meat Sauce	1 entree	6	290	550
Stuffed Cabbage With Whipped Potatoes	1 entree	7	220	460
Zucchini Lasagna	1 entree	4	240	470
STOUFFER'S® Entrees:				
Beef Pie	1 entree	26	450	1140
Beef Ravioli	1 entree	14	370	680
Cheese Manicotti	1 entree	16	340	810
Cheese Ravioli With Tomato Sauce	1 entree	14	360	720
Chicken Pie	1 entree	33	520	1000

Frozen, Canned, and Boxed Entrees and Meals

FOOD	SERVING SIZE	FAT GMS	CALS	NA MGS
Frozen Items (Continued):				
STOUFFER'S® Entrees (Continued):				
Four Cheese Lasagna	1 entree	19	410	840
Green Pepper Steak	1 entree	9	330	650
Homestyle Fried Chicken & Whipped Potatoes	1 entree	16	330	780
Homestyle Roast Turkey & Homestyle Stuffing	1 entree	11	280	950
Lasagna With Meat Sauce	1 entree	13	360	780
Macaroni & Cheese	1 entree	16	310	970
WEIGHT WATCHERS® Entrees:				
Barbecue Glazed Chicken	1 entree	4	190	340
Broccoli/Cheese Baked Potato	1 entree	7	230	510
Chicken Fettucini	1 entree	9	280	590
Deluxe Combo Pizza	1 pizza	11	380	550
Fettucini Alfredo & Broccoli	1 entree	6	220	540
Fried Fillet Of Fish	1 entree	8	230	450
Garden Lasagna	1 entree	5	230	460
Grilled Salisbury Steak	1 entree	9	250	590
Macaroni & Cheese	1 entree	6	260	550
Penne Pasta With Sun-Dried Tomatoes	1 entree	9	290	550
WEIGHT WATCHERS® Sandwiches *On-The-Go!:*				
Chicken, Broccoli & Cheddar Pocket	1 sandwich	6	250	310
Deluxe Pizza Pocket	1 sandwich	7	300	490
Grilled Chicken	1 sandwich	5	210	420
Reuben Pocket	1 sandwich	6	250	400
WEIGHT WATCHERS® SMART ONES™:				
Chicken Chow Mein	1 entree	2	200	430
Lasagna Florentine	1 entree	2	210	420
Lemon Herb Chicken Piccata	1 entree	2	190	590
Microwave Meals:				
CHEF BOYARDEE® Microwave Bowls:				
Beef Stew	1 bowl (7.5 oz.)	11	220	980
Lasagna With Pasta & Beef In Sauce	1 bowl (7.5 oz.)	8	230	880
Meat Tortellini With Beef In Tomato Sauce	1 bowl (7.5 oz.)	3	210	690
Pasta/Mini Meatballs In Tomato Sauce	1 bowl (7.5 oz.)	9	230	740
Ravioli, Beef In Tomato & Meat Sauce	1 bowl (7.5 oz.)	3	180	1040
Rice With Chicken/Vegetables	1 bowl (7.25 oz.)	6	220	830
Spaghetti & Meat Balls In Tomato Sauce	1 bowl (7.5 oz.)	6	200	870
CHEF BOYARDEE® Main Meals Microwave Bowls:				
Classic Noodles & Chicken With Vegetables	1 bowl (10.5 oz.)	1	170	1190
Meat Tortellini With Beef In Tomato Sauce	1 bowl (10.5 oz.)	4	300	980
Ziti Macaroni/Tomato Sauce	1 bowl (10.5 oz.)	0	240	1020
DINTY MOORE® Microwave Cups:				
Beef Stew	1 cup	10	190	870
Chicken & Dumpling	1 cup	6	190	670
Corned Beef Hash	1 cup	22	350	850

Frozen, Canned, and Boxed Entrees and Meals

FOOD	SERVING SIZE	FAT GMS	CALS	NA MGS
HORMEL® Micro Cup Meals:				
Beef Stew	1 cup	9	180	880
Lasagna	1 cup	7	230	650
Macaroni & Beef/Vegetables	1 cup	8	290	920
Macaroni & Cheese	1 cup	11	260	690
Noodles & Chicken	1 cup	8	180	1010
Spaghetti & Meat Sauce	1 cup	5	220	670
Pizza, Frozen:				
PAPPALO'S®, Deep Dish:				
Supreme	1/5 pizza	14	340	680
Three Cheese	1/4 pizza	12	370	670
PAPPALO'S®, For One:				
Supreme	1 pizza	27	560	1170
Three Cheese	1 pizza	20	500	960
RED BARON®, Deep Dish Singles:				
Cheese	1 pizza	26	500	820
Sausage	1 pizza	29	520	900
RED BARON® Pizza:				
Four Cheese	1/5 pizza	17	350	680
Supreme	1/5 pizza	19	360	730
TOMBSTONE® LIGHT Pizza:				
Supreme	1/5 pizza	9	270	710
Vegetable	1/5 pizza	7	240	500
TONY'S® Italian Style Pastry Crust Pizza:				
Sausage	1/3 pizza	24	420	710
Garden Supreme	1/3 pizza	19	370	720
TONY'S® Personal Pizza:				
Cheese	1 pizza	29	570	1090
Supreme	1 pizza	38	660	1490
TONY'S® Personal French Bread Pizza:				
Cheese	1 pizza	9	310	970
Supreme	1 pizza	16	380	1200
TOTINO'S® Party Pizza®:				
Cheese	1/2 pizza	14	320	630
Hamburger	1/2 pizza	18	350	860
Supreme	1/2 pizza	20	380	890
TOTINO'S® Microwave Pizza For One:				
Cheese	1 pizza	11	240	530
Supreme	1 pizza	17	290	680
Sauces, Canned:				
GREEN GIANT®:				
Sloppy Joe Sandwich Sauce & Meat	1 serving	11	200	470
HUNT'S MANWICH®, Sauce Only:				
Original Manwich	1/4 cup	0	30	370
Burrito Manwich	1/4 cup	0	30	560
Barbecue Manwich	1/4 cup	0	60	890

Frozen, Canned, and Boxed Entrees and Meals

FREE FOODS

Unsalted Bouillon Cubes or Broth or Regular Bouillon or Broth, if Sodium Is Not a Concern
Seltzer Water (No Salt or Sodium)
Coffee, Black, Unsweetened
Coffee, Decaffeinated, Black, Unsweetened
"Diet" Carbonated Beverages
Low Sodium Dill Pickles
Most Flavoring Essences
Horseradish
Herbs
Low Sodium Mustard or Regular Mustard, if Sodium Is Not a Concern
Pan Sprays, Non Stick
Pimiento, Unsalted, Canned
Spices
Tabasco Sauce
Tea, Unsweetened
Vinegar

FOOD	SERVING SIZE	FAT GMS	CALS	NA MGS

FRANCHISE RESTAURANTS
APPLEBEE'S® Neighborhood Grill & Bar
Selected Menu Items, Low Fat:

FOOD	SERVING SIZE	FAT GMS	CALS	NA MGS
Lemon Herbed Chicken With Pasta	1 serving	12	560	?-
Blackened Chicken Salad	1 serving	5	460	?-
Chicken Fajita Quesadilla	1 serving	11	490	?-
Stir-Fry Chicken	1 serving	7	570	?-
Veggie Combo Platter With 1 Garlic Bread & Whipped Margarine	1 serving	28	530	?-
House Salad (No Dressing)	1 serving	18	300	?-
Bikini Banana Lowfat Strawberry Shortcake	1 serving	2	250	?-

ARBY'S®
Breakfast Items:

FOOD	SERVING SIZE	FAT GMS	CALS	NA MGS
Toastix	1 serving	25	420	440
Maple Syrup	1 serving	0	120	50
Cinnamon Nut Danish	1	11	360	110
Biscuit:				
Plain	1	15	280	730
Bacon	1	18	320	900
Sausage	1	32	460	1000
Ham	1	17	320	1170
Croissant:				
Plain	1	16	260	300
Bacon/Egg	1	30	430	720
Ham/Cheese	1	21	350	940
Mushroom/Cheese	1	38	490	940
Sausage/Egg	1	39	520	630
Platters:				
Ham	1	26	520	1180
Sausage	1	41	640	860
Egg	1	24	460	590
Bacon	1	33	590	880
Blueberry Muffin	1	7	240	200
Roast Beef Sandwiches:				
Regular	1	18	380	940
Beef 'N Cheddar	1	27	510	1170
Junior	1	11	230	520
Giant	1	26	540	1430
Super	1	28	550	1170
Philly Beef 'N Swiss	1	25	470	1140
Bac 'N Cheddar Deluxe	1	32	510	1090
French Dip	1	15	370	1020
French Dip 'N Swiss	1	19	430	1440
Arby Q	1	15	390	1270
Chicken Sandwiches:				
Breast Fillet	1	23	450	960
Roast Club	1	27	500	1140
Cordon Bleu	1	27	520	1460
Grilled Deluxe	1	20	430	900
Grilled Barbecue	1	13	390	1000

Applebee's and Arby's

FOOD	SERVING SIZE	FAT GMS	CALS	NA MGS
ARBY'S® (Continued)				
Other Sandwiches:				
Fish Fillet	1	27	530	870
Ham 'N Cheese	1	14	360	1400
Arby's Sub Shop:				
Italian Sub	1	39	670	2060
Roast Beef Sub	1	32	620	1850
Tuna Sub	1	37	660	1340
Turkey Sub	1	19	490	2030
Light Sandwiches:				
Roast Beef Deluxe	1	10	290	830
Roast Turkey Deluxe	1	6	260	1260
Roast Chicken Deluxe	1	7	280	780
Potatoes:				
French Fries	1 serving	13	250	110
Potato Cakes	1 serving	12	200	400
Curly Fries	1 serving	18	340	170
Cheddar Fries	1 serving	22	400	440
Baked:				
Plain	1	2	240	60
With Butter/Margarine & Sour Cream	1	25	460	200
Broccoli & Cheese	1	18	420	360
Deluxe	1	36	620	610
Mushroom 'N Cheese	1	27	520	920
Salads:				
Garden	1	5	120	130
Roast Chicken	1	7	200	510
Chef	1	10	210	800
Side	1	0	30	30
Salad Dressings:				
Honey French	1 serving	27	320	490
Light Italian	1 serving	1	20	1110
Thousand Island	1 serving	29	300	490
Blue Cheese	1 serving	31	300	490
Buttermilk Ranch	1 serving	39	350	470
Croutons	1 tablespoon	2	60	160
Soups:				
Boston Clam Chowder	1 serving	10	190	1030
Cream Of Broccoli	1 serving	7	170	1050
Lumberjack Mixed Vegetable	1 serving	4	90	1080
Old Fashioned Chicken Noodle	1 serving	2	100	930
Potato With Bacon	1 serving	9	180	1070
Wisconsin Cheese	1 serving	18	280	1080
Desserts:				
Apple Turnover	1	18	300	180
Cherry Turnover	1	18	280	200
Blueberry Turnover	1	19	320	240
Cheese Cake	1	23	300	220
Chocolate Chip Cookie	1	4	130	100
Chocolate Shake	1	12	450	340
Vanilla Shake	1	12	330	280
Jamocha Shake	1	11	370	260
Peanut Butter Cup Polar Swirl	1	24	520	390
Oreo Polar Swirl	1	20	480	520
Snickers Polar Swirl	1	19	510	350
Heath Polar Swirl	1	22	540	350
Butterfinger Polar Swirl	1	18	460	320

FOOD	SERVING SIZE	FAT GMS	CALS	NA MGS
ARBY'S® (Continued)				
Condiments:				
Arby's Sauce	1 serving	0	20	110
Horsey Sauce	1 serving	5	60	110
Ketchup	1 serving	0	20	140
Mustard	1 serving	1	10	160
Mayonnaise P.C.	1 serving	10	90	80
Au Jus	1 serving	0	10	750
BASKIN-ROBBINS®				
PRODUCTS ON THE LIGHTER SIDE:				
Hard Scooped:				
Chocolate Vanilla Twist	1/2 cup (4 oz.)	0	100	100
Daiquiri Ice	1 regular scoop	0	130	10
Red Raspberry Sorbet	1 regular scoop	0	140	10
Last Mango In Paradise Yogurt	1/2 cup (4 oz.)	0	130	70
Low Fat Ice Cream & Sherbets:				
Espresso 'N Cream	1/2 cup (4 oz.)	3	110	60
Rainbow Sherbet	1 regular scoop	2	160	40
LOW FAT YOGURT GONE CRAZY™:				
Maui Brownie Madness	1/2 cup (4 oz.)	3	140	80
Perils Of Praline	1/2 cup (4 oz.)	3	130	100
Raspberry Cheese Louise	1/2 cup (4 oz.)	3	130	100
No Sugar Added Ice Cream, With Aspartame & Sorbitol:				
Chocolate Chocolate Chip	1/2 cup (4 oz.)	3	100	70
Thin Mint	1/2 cup (4 oz.)	3	100	70
Soft Serve:				
Silk Chocolate	1/2 cup (4 oz.)	0	120	80
Vanilla Bean Dream	1/2 cup (4 oz.)	0	120	90
Dutch Chocolate Yogurt	1/2 cup (4 oz.)	0	100	60
Strawberry Yogurt	1/2 cup (4 oz.)	0	100	60
Vanilla Yogurt	1/2 cup (4 oz.)	0	110	70
TRULY FREE™ YOGURT GONE CRAZY™:				
Cafe Mocha	1/2 cup (4 oz.)	0	80	80
Chocolate	1/2 cup (4 oz.)	0	80	80
Vanilla	1/2 cup (4 oz.)	0	80	80
PREMIUM HARD SCOOPED ICE CREAM:				
Chocolate	1 regular scoop	16	270	110
Chocolate Chip	1 regular scoop	18	270	90
Rocky Road	1 regular scoop	17	300	110
Vanilla	1 regular scoop	14	240	70
Very Berry Strawberry	1 regular scoop	12	220	80
CAPPUCINNO BLAST™	16 ounces	10	280	110
BURGER KING®				
Burgers:				
Whopper	1	39	640	870
Whopper With Cheese	1	46	730	1300
Double Whopper	1	56	870	940
Double Whopper With Cheese	1	63	960	1360
Whopper Junior	1	24	420	570
Whopper Junior With Cheese	1	28	460	780
Cheeseburger	1	19	360	780
Double Cheeseburger	1	36	600	1040
Double Cheeseburger & Bacon	1	39	640	1220
Hamburger	1	15	330	570

FOOD	SERVING SIZE	FAT GMS	CALS	NA MGS
BURGER KING® (Continued)				
Sandwiches And Side Orders:				
BK Big Fish Sandwich	1	43	720	1090
BK Broiler Chicken Sandwich	1	29	540	480
Chicken Sandwich	1	43	700	1400
Chicken Tenders	6 pieces	12	250	530
Broiled Chicken Salad, No Dressing	1	10	200	110
Garden Salad, No Dressing	1	5	90	110
Side Salad, No Dressing	1	3	50	60
French Fries, Medium, Salted	1 serving	20	400	240
Onion Rings	1 serving	14	310	810
Dutch Apple Pie	1 serving	15	310	230
Drinks:				
Vanilla Shake	1 medium	7	310	230
Chocolate Shake	1 medium	7	310	230
Chocolate Shake/Syrup Added	1 medium	7	460	300
Strawberry Shake/Syrup Added	1 medium	7	430	260
Coca-Cola Classic	1 medium	0	260	?-
Sprite	1 medium	0	260	?-
Breakfast:				
Croissan'wich:				
With Bacon, Egg & Cheese	1	24	350	790
With Sausage, Egg & Cheese	1	41	530	1000
With Ham, Egg & Cheese	1	22	350	1390
French Toast Sticks	1 serving	27	500	490
Hash Browns	1 serving	12	220	320
Condiments & Toppings:				
Mayonnaise	1 serving	23	210	160
Tartar Sauce	1 serving	19	180	220
LAND O' LAKES® Whipped Cheese Blend	1 serving	7	70	80
Bull's Eye Barbecue Sauce	1 serving	0	20	140
Bacon Bits	1 serving	1	20	?-
Croutons	1 serving	1	30	80
NEWMAN'S OWN® Salad Dressings:				
Thousand Island	1 serving	12	140	190
French	1 serving	10	140	190
Ranch	1 serving	19	180	170
Blue Cheese	1 serving	16	160	260
Reduced Calorie Light Italian	1 serving	1	20	50
Dipping Sauces:				
A.M. Express	1 serving	0	80	20
Honey Express	1 serving	0	90	10
Ranch	1 serving	17	170	200
Barbecue	1 serving	0	40	400
Sweet & Sour	1 serving	0	50	50
CAPTAIN D'S®				
Broiled & Baked Dinners (Includes Rice, Green Beans, Bread Stick, Salad And Low Calorie Italian Dressing):				
Orange Roughy Dinner	1	19	540	2160
Shrimp Dinner	1	10	460	2190
Chicken Dinner	1	8	410	2620
Baked Fish Dinner (With Cole Slaw, Not Salad)	1	18	550	1180

Burger King and Captain D's

FOOD	SERVING SIZE	FAT GMS	CALS	NA MGS
CAPTAIN D'S® (Continued)				
Sandwich:				
Broiled Chicken	1 sandwich	19	450	860
Side Items:				
Stuffed Crab	1 serving	7	90	250
Cracklins	1 ounce	17	220	740
French Fried Potatoes	1 serving	10	300	150
Cole Slaw	1 serving	12	160	250
Cole Slaw	1 pint	47	630	450
Cob Corn	1 serving	2	250	10
Baked Potato	1 serving	0	280	20
Green Beans, Seasoned	1 serving	2	50	750
White Beans	1 serving	1	130	100
Rice	1 serving	0	120	10
Fried Okra	1 serving	16	300	450
Hushpuppy	1	4	130	470
Hushpuppies	6	25	760	2790
Breadstick	1	1	90	210
Breadsticks	6	7	550	1260
Dinner Salad, No Dressing	1 serving	1	30	70
Dressings:				
French	1 packet	11	110	190
Blue Cheese	1 packet	12	110	100
Ranch	1 packet	10	90	230
Low Calorie Italian	1 packet	1	20	440
Crackers	4 crackers	1	50	150
Slice of Cheese	1 slice	5	50	210
Cocktail Sauce	1 side portion	0	30	250
Cocktail Sauce	1 bulk portion	0	140	1010
Tartar Sauce	1 side portion	7	80	160
Tartar Sauce	1 bulk portion	27	300	630
Sweet & Sour Sauce	1 side portion	0	50	10
Sweet & Sour Sauce	1 bulk portion	0	210	20
Nondairy Creamer	2 creamers	2	30	20
Desserts:				
Pecan Pie	1 piece	20	460	370
Chocolate Cake	1 piece	10	300	260
Carrot Cake	1 piece	23	430	410
Cheesecake	1 piece	31	420	480
Lemon Pie	1 piece	10	350	140
CHURCH'S® FRIED CHICKEN				
Chicken:				
Wing	1 serving	16	250	540
Leg	1 serving	9	140	160
Thigh	1 serving	16	230	520
Breast	1 serving	12	200	510
Sides:				
Cajun Rice	1 serving	7	130	260
Potatoes 'N Gravy	1 serving	3	90	520
Okra	1 serving	16	210	520
Biscuits	1 serving	16	250	640
Corn On The Cob	1 serving	3	140	20
Coleslaw	1 serving	6	90	230
French Fries	1 serving	11	210	60
Apple Pie	1 serving	12	280	340

Captain D's and Church's Fried Chicken

FOOD	SERVING SIZE	FAT GMS	CALS	NA MGS
COUNTRY KITCHEN® RIGHT CHOICE™				
Breakfast:				
Blueberry Pancakes	1 serving	12	360	?-
Best Cakes In Town	1 full stack	12	430	?-
Best Cakes In Town	1 short stack	10	370	?-
Garden Omelet	1 serving	6	370	?-
Healthy Egg Breakfast With Fruit, Dry Toast & Jelly	1 serving	5	310	?-
Hot Or Cold Cereal With Fruit, 2% Milk, Dry Toast & Jelly	1 serving	6	470	?-
Entrees:				
Beef & Broccoli Stir Fry	1 serving	18	530	?-
Chicken Stir Fry	1 serving	10	420	?-
Oriental Chicken & Fried Rice	1 serving	15	470	?-
Herb Grilled Chicken & Fresh Tomato Pasta	1 serving	15	740	?-
Grilled Chicken Dinner	1 serving	9	290	?-
Chicken Stir Fry Pita	1 serving	3	390	?-
Side Dishes:				
Applesauce	1 serving	0	90	?-
Glazed Baby Carrots	1 serving	3	100	?-
Dinner Salad With Reduced Calorie Dressing	1 serving	8	170	?-
Baked Potato & Sour Cream	1 serving	6	280	?-
Rice Pilaf	1 serving	1	70	?-
Cup Calico Bean Soup	1 serving	4	130	?-
Vegetable Of The Day	1 serving	6	110	?-
Cottage Cheese	1 serving	2	110	?-
Sandwiches And Salads:				
Grilled Chicken Salad & Dinner Roll	1 serving	23	620	?-
Soup & Salad	1 serving	14	360	?-
Grilled Chicken Breast Salad	1 serving	21	530	?-
French Dip Sandwich	1 serving	19	650	?-
Philly Beef And Cheese Sandwich	1 serving	27	850	?-
DAIRY QUEEN®				
Blizzards:				
Strawberry, Small	1 serving	12	400	160
Strawberry, Regular	1 serving	16	570	230
Heath, Small	1 serving	23	560	280
Heath, Regular	1 serving	36	820	410
Breezes:				
Strawberry, Small	1 serving	0	290	120
Strawberry, Regular	1 serving	1	420	170
Heath, Small	1 serving	12	450	230
Heath, Regular	1 serving	21	680	360
Cones:				
Vanilla, Small	1 cone	4	140	60
Vanilla, Regular	1 cone	7	230	100
Vanilla, Large	1 cone	10	340	140
Chocolate, Regular	1 cone	7	230	120
Chocolate, Large	1 cone	11	350	170
Chocolate, Regular, Dipped	1 cone	16	330	100
Yogurt, Regular	1 cone	0	180	80
Yogurt, Large	1 cone	0	260	120

FOOD	SERVING SIZE	FAT GMS	CALS	NA MGS
DAIRY QUEEN® (Continued)				
Cups And Scoops:				
DQ Vanilla, Big	1 scoop	14	300	100
DQ Chocolate, Big	1 scoop	14	310	100
Yogurt, Regular	1 cup	0	170	70
Yogurt, Large	1 cup	0	230	100
Miscellaneous Desserts:				
Banana Split	1	11	510	250
Buster Bar	1	29	460	220
Dilly Bar	1	13	210	50
DQ Sandwich	1	4	140	140
DQ Frozen Cake Slice	1	18	380	210
Hot Fudge Brownie Delight	1	29	710	340
Nutty Double Fudge	1	22	580	170
Peanut Buster Parfait	1	32	710	410
Mr. Misty, Regular	1 serving	0	250	0
Shakes:				
Vanilla, Regular	1	14	520	230
Vanilla, Large	1	16	600	260
Chocolate, Regular	1	14	540	290
Vanilla Malt, Regular	1	14	610	230
Sundaes:				
Chocolate, Regular	1 serving	7	300	140
Strawberry Waffle Cone	1 serving	12	350	220
Strawberry Yogurt, Regular	1 serving	0	200	80
Sandwiches:				
Hamburger:				
Single	1	13	310	580
Single With Cheese	1	18	370	800
Double	1	25	460	630
Double With Cheese	1	34	570	1070
DQ Homestyle, Ultimate	1	47	700	1110
Hot Dog:				
Regular	1	16	280	700
With Cheese	1	21	330	920
With Chili	1	19	320	720
1/4# Super Dog	1	38	590	1360
BBQ Beef	1	9	300	?-
Grilled Chicken Fillet	1	8	300	800
Breaded Chicken Fillet:				
Regular	1	20	430	760
With Cheese	1	25	480	980
Fish Fillet:				
Regular	1	16	370	630
With Cheese	1	21	420	850
Salads:				
Side, No Dressing	1 serving	0	30	10
Garden, No Dressing	1 serving	13	200	240
Salad Dressings:				
Thousand Island	1 serving	21	230	570
Reduced Calorie French	1 serving	5	90	450
French Fries:				
Small	1 serving	10	210	120
Regular	1 serving	14	300	160
Large	1 serving	18	390	200
Onion Rings, Regular	1 serving	12	240	140

Dairy Queen

FOOD	SERVING SIZE	FAT GMS	CALS	NA MGS
DENNY'S®				
Daybreaks:				
Slams:				
All American (No Bread)	1 serving	84	980	1500
French	1 serving	60	920	1090
Grand Slam	1 serving	45	860	2100
Harvest	1 serving	56	1060	2200
International	1 serving	68	980	1050
Scram (No Bread)	1 serving	91	1080	2070
Southern	1 serving	71	900	2230
Omelettes (Omelette Only):				
Chili Cheese	1 serving	33	450	870
Denver	1 serving	63	740	920
Ham 'N Cheddar	1 serving	34	490	1150
Mexican	1 serving	41	550	1090
Senior	1 serving	58	650	1360
Ultimate	1 serving	64	750	1250
Vegetable	1 serving	48	590	530
Breakfast Favorites:				
Chicken Fried Steak & Eggs (No Bread)	1 serving	49	650	1270
Moons Over My Hammy	1 serving	66	980	3160
Steak & Eggs (No Bread)	1 serving	51	800	740
Griddle Favorites:				
Belgian Waffle	1 serving	22	320	230
Buttermilk Pancakes	3 plain	6	410	1970
French Toast	1 serving	19	330	310
Griddle Favorite Toppings:				
Blueberry Topping	6 tablespoons	0	110	20
Strawberry Topping	6 tablespoons	0	80	10
Whipped Topping	4 tablespoons	2	20	10
Syrup	4 tablespoons	0	160	50
Whipped Butter	1 tablespoon	7	70	80
Breakfast Sides:				
Applesauce	1 serving (1/4 cup)	0	40	10
Bacon	4 strips	12	150	410
Bagel	1	1	230	540
Banana	1	1	110	0
Banana Strawberry Medley	1 serving	0	100	0
Biscuit, Plain	1 biscuit	9	220	80
Biscuit With Sausage Gravy	1 serving	30	470	1490
Blueberry Muffin	1 muffin	14	310	190
Cantaloupe	1/4	0	100	60
Cinnamon Roll	1	30	670	400
Cream Cheese	1 ounce	10	100	40
Egg	1	10	120	200
English Muffin	1 muffin	1	150	410
Grapefruit	1/2	0	40	0
Grapes	1 serving	0	60	0
Grits	1 serving	0	160	880
Ham	1 serving	8	170	850
Hash Browns	1 serving	13	210	430
Honey Dew	1/4	0	130	40
Orange Juice	10 ounces	0	130	0
Sausage	4 links	22	230	390
Toast, Dry	2 pieces	2	140	200

FOOD	SERVING SIZE	FAT GMS	CALS	NA MGS
DENNY'S® (Continued)				
Salads:				
Caesar Salad	1 serving	23	330	590
California Grilled Chicken	1 serving	12	290	550
Chef's Salad	1 serving	26	370	1340
Crispy Chicken Salad	1 serving	55	910	1810
Crispy Chicken Salad, Without Tortilla Shell	1 serving	25	470	1200
Garden Salad	1 serving	4	120	160
Grilled Chicken Caesar Salad	1 serving	41	660	1260
Taco Salad	1 serving	55	910	1850
Taco Salad, Without Shell	1 serving	25	470	1250
Salad Dressings:				
Bleu Cheese	2 tablespoons	14	120	440
Creamy Italian	2 tablespoons	10	100	340
French	2 tablespoons	12	100	400
French Reduced Calorie	2 tablespoons	4	70	370
Honey Mustard	2 tablespoons	6	100	220
Italian Reduced Calorie	2 tablespoons	1	20	380
Ranch	2 tablespoons	11	110	190
1000 Island	2 tablespoons	11	120	220
Sandwiches:				
Bacon Lettuce & Tomato	1 serving	37	490	830
Chicken Melt	1 serving	41	700	1430
Club	1 serving	35	490	1390
French Dip	1 serving	40	580	1590
Grilled Cheese	1 serving	49	720	2390
Grilled Chicken	1 serving	34	670	1300
MegaMelt	1 serving	63	950	3110
Prime Time	1 serving	70	930	1890
Roast Beef Deluxe	1 serving	56	850	1740
Super Bird	1 serving	35	590	1860
Tuna Melt Supreme	1 serving	58	810	2090
Veggie Cheese Melt	1 serving	40	570	1350
Burgers:				
Bacon-Swiss	1 serving	45	750	1460
Denny Burger	1 serving	25	490	480
Patty Melt	1 serving	58	780	1410
Works Burger	1 serving	66	950	1370
Sides:				
Coleslaw	1 serving	9	110	40
French Fries	1 serving	12	290	120
Soups:				
Cheese	1 serving	23	320	900
Chicken Noodle	1 serving	2	60	650
Chili With Beans	1 serving	6	160	680
Clam Chowder	1 serving	12	220	900
Cream Of Broccoli	1 serving	12	200	820
Cream Of Potato	1 serving	12	230	760
Vegetable Beef	1 serving	1	80	830
Starters:				
Buffalo Wings, No Dressing	1 serving	22	350	1570
Chicken Strips, No Dressing	1 serving	25	580	1340
Chili Fries	1 serving	25	585	650
Mozzarella Sticks	1 serving (4)	20	350	830
Nachos Supreme	1 serving	45	770	1320
Quesadilla	1 serving	28	460	1590
Chicken Quesadilla	1 serving	31	580	1970

FOOD	SERVING SIZE	FAT GMS	CALS	NA MGS
DENNY'S® (Continued)				
Entrees:				
Chicken Fried Steak	1 serving	38	470	1400
Chicken Strips	1 serving	25	580	1340
Fried Chicken	1 serving	27	460	1660
Grilled Breast Of Chicken	1 serving (4 oz.)	3	130	390
Grilled Breast Of Chicken	1 serving (6 oz.)	5	190	580
Grilled Catfish	1 serving	43	480	90
Grilled Rainbow Trout	1 serving	34	490	520
Liver With Bacon & Onions	1 serving	41	590	320
Prime Rib	1 serving (8 oz.)	46	570	1180
Roast Beef & Bread, Potatoes/ Gravy	1 serving	19	600	820
Roast Turkey/Stuffing & Gravy	1 serving	26	490	1750
Spaghetti With Meatballs	1 serving	38	1000	2030
Spaghetti With Sauce	1 serving	9	610	950
Stir Fry Chicken/Vegetables & Rice Pilaf	1 serving	21	440	1020
Desserts:				
Chocolate Cake	1 serving	17	370	360
Banana Split	1 serving	37	850	280
Double Dip Sundae	1 serving	26	550	160
Hot Fudge Cake Sundae	1 serving	39	730	500
Hot Fudge Sundae	1 serving	30	500	200
Ice Cream	1 scoop	7	140	60
Ice Cream Shake	1 serving	24	530	250
Pies:				
Apple	1 serving	30	520	280
Apple With EQUAL®	1 serving	30	460	200
Blueberry Cream Cheese	1 serving	37	700	500
Cherry	1 serving	30	640	320
Cherry With Equal	1 serving	30	510	170
Cherry Cream Cheese	1 serving	37	690	500
Chocolate Cream	1 serving	30	510	340
Coconut Cream	1 serving	27	480	370
Key Lime	1 serving	27	590	190
SENIOR SELECTIONS:				
Senior Breakfast Items:				
Senior Belgian Waffle Slam	1 serving	46	540	710
Syrup	1 serving (1/4 cup)	0	160	50
Senior Grand Slam	1 serving	24	540	1160
Senior Omelette	1 serving	57	640	1340
Senior Starter	1 serving	45	550	920
Senior Lunch & Dinner Entrees:				
(Vegetable Choice Not Included)				
Senior Catfish Dinner	1 serving	32	450	530
Senior Chicken Fried Steak	1 serving	23	430	1190
Senior Fried Chicken	1 serving	23	480	1830
Senior Grilled Cheese Sandwich	1 serving	25	360	1190
Senior Grilled Chicken Dinner	1 serving	7	250	810
Senior Liver/Bacon & Onions	1 serving	27	440	660
Senior Roast Beef	1 serving	9	280	520
Senior Roast Turkey & Stuffing	1 serving	16	440	950
Senior Sirloin Tips	1 serving	5	220	680
Senior Spaghetti & Meatballs	1 serving	25	580	1010
Senior Tuna Salad Sandwich	1 serving	17	260	420
Senior Turkey Sandwich	1 serving	27	340	1000

FOOD	SERVING SIZE	FAT GMS	CALS	NA MGS
EL POLLO LOCO®				
Chicken:				
Breast	1	6	160	390
Leg	1	5	90	150
Thigh	1	12	180	230
Wing	1	6	110	220
Tortillas:				
Corn	1	1	60	30
Flour	1	3	90	150
Side Dishes:				
Beans	1 serving	3	100	460
Rice	1 serving	2	110	220
Corn	1 serving	2	110	110
Potato Salad	1 serving	10	180	340
Coleslaw	1 serving	8	100	160
Salads:				
Side Salad, No Dressing	1 serving	1	50	30
Chicken Salad, No Dressing	1 serving	4	160	440
Tacos, Burritos & Fajitas:				
Bean, Rice & Cheese Burrito	1 serving	13	530	730
Vegetarian Burrito	1 serving	7	340	360
Chicken Burrito	1 serving	11	310	510
Classic Chicken Burrito	1 serving	20	560	1170
Spicy Hot Chicken Burrito	1 serving	20	570	1180
Whole Wheat Chicken Burrito	1 serving	16	510	900
Loco Grande Chicken Burrito	1 serving	30	680	1290
Steak Burrito	1 serving	22	450	740
Grilled Steak Burrito	1 serving	29	740	1180
Steak Fajita Meal	1 serving	38	1040	1550
Chicken Fajita Meal	1 serving	18	780	1060
Chicken Taco	1 serving	7	180	300
Steak Taco	1 serving	12	250	410
Condiments:				
Cheddar Cheese	1 oz.	5	90	180
Guacamole	1 oz.	6	60	130
Salsa	1 oz.	0	10	180
Sour Cream	1 oz.	6	60	20
Honey Dijon Mustard	1 oz.	1	50	440
Deluxe French Dressing	1 oz.	4	60	160
1000 Island Dressing	1 oz.	10	110	240
Reduced Calorie Italian Dressing	1 oz.	2	30	170
Ranch Dressing	1 oz.	6	80	190
Blue Cheese Dressing	1 oz.	6	80	150
Desserts:				
Cheesecake	1 serving	18	310	230
Churro	1 serving	8	130	160

FOOD	SERVING SIZE	FAT GMS	CALS	NA MGS
GODFATHER'S PIZZA®				
Original Crust:				
Cheese Pizza:				
Mini	1/4 pizza	4	140	160
Small	1/6 pizza	7	240	290
Medium	1/8 pizza	7	240	290
Large	1/10 pizza	8	270	330
Combo Pizza:				
Mini	1/4 pizza	5	160	290
Small	1/6 pizza	11	300	570
Medium	1/8 pizza	12	320	570
Large	1/10 pizza	12	330	620
Golden Crust:				
Cheese Pizza:				
Small	1/6 pizza	8	210	260
Medium	1/8 pizza	9	230	270
Large	1/10 pizza	11	260	310
Combo Pizza:				
Small	1/6 pizza	12	270	540
Medium	1/8 pizza	13	280	530
Large	1/10 pizza	15	320	600
HARDEES®				
Breakfast Menu:				
BISCUIT:				
RISE 'N' SHINE™	1	21	390	1000
CINNAMON 'N' RAISIN™	1	18	370	450
Sausage	1	31	510	1360
Sausage & Egg	1	35	560	1400
Bacon & Egg	1	27	490	1250
Bacon, Egg & Cheese	1	31	530	1470
Ham	1	20	400	1340
Ham, Egg & Cheese	1	27	500	1620
Country Ham	1	22	430	1930
CANADIAN RISE 'N' SHINE™	1	32	570	1860
Steak	1	32	580	1580
Chicken Fillet	1	25	510	1580
BIG COUNTRY BISCUIT™:				
Sausage	1	61	930	2240
Bacon	1	43	740	1800
FRISCO™ Breakfast Sandwich, Ham	1	22	460	1320
HASH ROUNDS™, Regular	1 serving	14	230	560
BISCUIT 'N' GRAVY™	1 serving	28	510	1500
Blueberry Muffin	1	17	400	310
Pancakes & Accompaniments:				
Three	1 serving	2	280	890
Three With Sausage Patty	1 serving	16	430	1290
Three With 2 Bacon Strips	1 serving	9	350	1130
Sandwiches:				
Hamburgers:				
Plain	1	9	260	460
Cheeseburger	1	13	300	690
Quarter-Pound With Cheese	1	25	490	860
BIG DELUXE™	1	30	530	790

FOOD	SERVING SIZE	FAT GMS	CALS	NA MGS
HARDEES® (Continued)				
Burgers (Continued):				
Bacon & Cheese	1	36	600	950
MUSHROOM 'N' SWISS™	1	27	520	990
FRISCO™ Burger	1	50	760	1280
Other Sandwiches:				
Roast Beef, Regular	1	11	270	780
BIG ROAST BEEF™	1	16	370	1050
HOT HAM 'N' CHEESE™	1	30	530	1710
FISHERMAN'S FILLET™	1	22	500	1170
Chicken Fillet	1	14	400	1100
FRISCO™ Grilled Chicken	1	34	620	1730
Hot Dog	1	20	450	1090
French Fries:				
Small	1 serving	10	240	100
Medium	1 serving	15	350	150
Large	1 serving	18	430	190
CRISPY CURLS™	1 serving	16	300	840
Side Items:				
Baked Beans, Small	1 serving	1	180	560
Baked Beans, Large	1 serving	4	530	1670
Baked Potato	1 serving	0	220	20
Sour Cream	1 serving	8	90	20
Green Beans, Small	1 serving	3	80	250
Green Beans, Large	1 serving	8	250	750
Macaroni 'N' Cheese, Small	1 serving	8	190	920
Macaroni 'N' Cheese, Large	1 serving	25	580	2770
Salads, No Dressing:				
Side	1	0	30	50
Garden	1	13	210	350
Grilled Chicken	1	3	150	610
Super Chef	1	12	230	800
Salad Dressings:				
Fat Free French	1 serving	0	70	580
Ranch	1 serving	29	290	510
Thousand Island	1 serving	23	250	540
Parmesan Peppercorn	1 serving	34	330	560
Fat Free Honey Dijon	1 serving	0	80	290
Italian	1 serving	24	230	430
Shakes And Desserts:				
Shakes:				
Vanilla	1	5	350	300
Chocolate	1	5	370	270
Strawberry	1	4	420	270
Peach	1	4	390	290
COOL TWIST™ Cones:				
Vanilla	1	2	170	130
Chocolate	1	2	180	110
Vanilla/Chocolate	1	2	180	120
COOL TWIST™ Sundaes:				
Hot Fudge	1	6	290	310
Strawberry	1	2	210	140
BIG COOKIE™	1	12	280	150

Hardee's

FOOD	SERVING SIZE	FAT GMS	CALS	NA MGS
JACK IN THE BOX®				
Breakfast:				
Breakfast Jack	1	12	300	890
Pancake Platter	1	22	610	890
Sausage Crescent	1	43	580	1010
Sausage Egg Platter	1	32	560	1060
Scrambled Egg Pocket	1	21	430	1060
Sourdough Breakfast Sandwich	1	20	380	1120
Supreme Crescent	1	33	530	930
Ultimate Breakfast Sandwich	1	35	620	1800
Hash Browns	1 serving	11	160	310
Country Crock Spread	1 serving	3	30	40
Grape Jelly	1 serving	0	40	0
Pancake Syrup	1 serving	0	120	0
Sandwiches:				
Chicken Caesar	1	26	520	1050
Chicken Fajita Pita	1	8	290	700
Chicken	1	18	400	1290
Chicken Supreme	1	36	620	1520
Country Fried Steak	1	25	450	890
Fish Supreme	1	32	590	1170
Grilled Chicken Fillet	1	19	430	1070
Monterey Roast Beef	1	30	540	1270
Smoked Chicken/Cheddar & Bacon	1	30	540	1520
Sourdough Ranch Chicken	1	21	490	1060
Spicy Crispy Chicken	1	27	560	1020
Hamburgers:				
Hamburger	1	11	280	430
Cheeseburger	1	15	330	510
Double Cheeseburger	1	24	450	900
Jumbo Jack	1	32	560	700
Jumbo Jack With Cheese	1	36	610	780
Bacon Bacon Cheeseburger	1	45	710	1240
Grilled Sourdough Burger	1	43	670	1140
Ultimate Cheeseburger	1	57	830	1180
Burger	1 (1/4 lb.)	27	510	1030
Colossus Burger	1	60	940	1670
Salads & Salad Dressings:				
Grilled Chicken Salad	1	9	200	420
Side Salad	1	4	70	80
Bleu Cheese Dressing	1 serving	18	210	750
Buttermilk House Dressing	1 serving	30	290	560
Low Calorie Italian Dressing	1 serving	2	30	670
1000 Island Dressing	1 serving	24	250	570
Croutons	1 serving	2	50	110
Mexican Food:				
Taco	1	11	190	410
Super Taco	1	17	280	720
Guacamole	1 serving	4	50	100
Salsa	1 serving	0	10	200
Finger Foods:				
Egg Rolls	3 pieces	24	440	960
Egg Rolls	5 pieces	41	750	1640
Chicken Strips, Breaded	4 pieces	13	290	700
Chicken Strips, Breaded	6 pieces	20	450	1100
Chicken Taquitos	5 pieces	15	350	570

FOOD	SERVING SIZE	FAT GMS	CALS	NA MGS
JACK IN THE BOX® (Continued)				
Chicken Taquitas	8 pieces	25	560	900
Barbeque Sauce	1 serving	0	50	300
Buttermilk House Sauce	1 serving	13	130	240
Hot Sauce	1 serving	0	10	110
Sweet & Sour Sauce	1 serving	0	40	160
Sides:				
Seasoned Curly Fries	1 serving	20	360	1070
Small French Fries	1 serving	11	220	120
Regular French Fries	1 serving	17	350	190
Jumbo Fries	1 serving	19	400	220
Super Scoop French Fries	1 serving	29	590	330
Onion Rings	1 serving	23	380	450
Desserts:				
Hot Apple Turnover	1	19	350	460
Cheesecake	1 serving	18	310	210
Chocolate Chip Cookie Dough Cheesecake	1 serving	18	360	200
Cinnamon Churritos	1 serving	21	330	200
KENNY ROGERS ROASTERS®				
Kenny's Smart Heart Meals:				
1/4 Chicken, White, Mashed Potatoes/Gravy, Corn Muffin	1 meal	11	410	940
1/4 Chicken, White, Rice Pilaf, Steamed Vegetables, Corn Muffin	1 meal	13	480	670
BBQ Chicken Pita, Side Salad	1 meal	7	380	920
Chicken Entrees:				
Chicken, White, With Skin	1 (1/4 chicken)	10	250	630
Chicken, White, No Skin	1 (1/4 chicken)	2	150	330
Chicken, Dark, With Skin	1 (1/4 chicken)	13	240	570
Chicken, Dark, No Skin	1 (1/4 chicken)	8	180	380
Chicken, With Skin	1 (1/2 chicken)	23	490	1200
Chicken, No Skin	1 (1/2 chicken)	10	330	710
Chicken, With Skin	1 whole	45	980	2390
Chicken, No Skin	1 whole	20	660	1420
Pitas & Pot Pie:				
BBQ Chicken Pita	1	7	360	900
Chicken Caesar Pita	1	32	570	1600
Roasted Chicken Pita	1	33	590	1530
Chicken Pot Pie	1	36	820	1770
Soups & Salads:				
Chicken Noodle Soup	1 cup	3	110	720
Chicken Noodle Soup	1 bowl	4	170	1150
Chicken Caesar Salad	1 serving	39	590	1220
Roasted Chicken Salad	1 serving	13	360	640
Side Dishes:				
Cinnamon Apples	1 serving	5	200	0
Cole Slaw	1 serving	16	230	290
Corn Muffins	1	6	110	160
Corn On The Cob	1	1	70	10
Garlic Parsley Potatoes	1 serving	12	260	870
Honey Baked Beans	1 serving	2	150	520
Macaroni & Cheese	1 serving	6	200	660
Mashed Potatoes & Gravy	1 serving	2	150	440
Pasta Salad	1 serving	17	270	420
Potato Salad	1 serving	27	390	630

Jack in The Box and Kenny Roger's Roasters

FOOD	SERVING SIZE	FAT GMS	CALS	NA MGS
KENNY ROGERS ROASTERS® (Continued)				
Side Dishes (Continued):				
Rice Pilaf	1 serving	5	170	150
Side Salad, No Dressing	1 serving	0	20	20
Steamed Vegetables	1 serving	0	50	60
Tomato Cucumber Salad	1 serving	10	130	520
Salad Dressings:				
Blue Cheese	1 serving	39	370	720
Buttermilk Ranch	1 serving	48	430	620
Caesar	1 serving	36	340	780
Dijon Honey Mustard	1 serving	28	320	410
Fat Free Italian	1 serving	0	40	1040
Honey French	1 serving	29	350	490
1000 Island	1 serving	33	330	550

KFC® (Kentucky Fried Chicken)

FOOD	SERVING SIZE	FAT GMS	CALS	NA MGS
Original Recipe Chicken:				
Wing	1 piece	8	150	380
Breast	1 piece	20	360	870
Drumstick	1 piece	7	130	210
Thigh	1 piece	17	260	570
Extra Tasty Crispy Chicken:				
Wing	1 piece	13	200	290
Breast	1 piece	28	470	930
Drumstick	1 piece	11	190	260
Thigh	1 piece	25	370	540
Rotisserie Gold:				
Breast & Wing Quarter	1 serving	19	340	1100
Thigh & Leg Quarter	1 serving	24	330	980
Hot & Spicy Chicken:				
Wing	1 piece	15	210	340
Breast	1 piece	35	530	1110
Drumstick	1 piece	11	190	300
Thigh	1 piece	27	370	570
Sides:				
Biscuit	1	12	200	560
Cornbread	1 serving	6	180	290
BBQ Baked Beans	1 serving	2	130	540
Corn-On-The-Cob	1 serving	12	220	80
Garden Rice	1 serving	1	80	580
Green Beans	1 serving	1	40	560
Mashed Potatoes & Gravy	1 serving	5	110	390
Mean Greens	1 serving	2	50	480
Potato Wedges	1 serving	9	190	430
Macaroni & Cheese	1 serving	8	160	530
Red Beans & Rice	1 serving	3	110	320
Coleslaw	1 serving	6	110	180
Potato Salad	1 serving	11	180	420
Snackables:				
Colonel's Chicken Sandwich	1	27	480	1060
Hot Wings	1 serving (6)	33	470	1230
Value BBQ Chicken Sandwich	1	8	260	780
Kentucky Nuggets	1 serving (6)	18	280	870

FOOD	SERVING SIZE	FAT GMS	CALS	NA MGS
LITTLE CAESAR'S PIZZA®				
Cheese Pizza, Round:				
Small Round	1/6	7	190	270
Medium Round	1/8	7	200	280
Large Round	1/10	8	210	310
Cheese Pan Pizza:				
Small Pan	1/6	6	190	390
Medium Pan	1/9	6	180	380
Large Pan	1/12	6	190	390
Pepperoni Pizza, Round:				
Small Round	1/6	8	210	350
Medium Round	1/8	9	220	360
Large Round	1/10	10	230	400
Pepperoni Pan Pizza:				
Small Pan	1/6	8	200	460
Medium Pan	1/9	8	200	450
Large Pan	1/12	8	200	460
Baby Pan! Pan!	1 (9.5 oz.)	24	620	1470
Slice Slice	1 (12 oz.)	34	800	1390
Crazy Bread	1	3	110	110
Crazy Sauce	1 serving	0	70	380
Spaghetti, Little Bucket	1 (approx. 1 #)	12	530	810
Lasagna	1 (approx. 1 #)	37	720	1610
Veal Parmigiana	1 portion	23	510	1040
Spaghetti	1 portion	6	260	400
Chocolate Ravioli	1	9	140	40
Sandwiches:				
Ham & Cheese	1	37	670	1460
Italian	1	43	720	1610
Tuna	1	38	730	1300
Turkey	1	23	560	1920
Vegetarian	1	54	870	1980
Big Veal Deal	1	26	530	910
Chicken	1	25	530	1040
Salads:				
Antipasto	1 serving	12	180	540
Caesar, No Dressing	1 serving	5	140	370
Tossed, No Dressing	1 serving	3	120	170
Greek	1 serving	10	170	650
LONG JOHN SILVER'S®				
Flavorbaked Meals:				
Flavorbaked Fish (2), Rice With Baked Potato & Green Beans	1 meal	10	520	?-
Flavorbaked Fish (2) Over Rice With Side Salad	1 meal	9	350	?-
Flavorbaked Chicken (1), Rice With Baked Potato & Green Beans	1 meal	8	450	?-
Flavorbaked Chicken (1), Rice With Side Salad	1 meal	7	280	?-
Flavorbaked Combination (1 Fish, 1 Chicken), Rice With Baked Potato & Green Beans	1 meal	10	540	?-
Sandwiches:				
Batter-Dipped Fish	1 sandwich	13	340	890
Batter-Dipped Chicken	1 sandwich	8	280	790
Flavorbaked Fish	1 sandwich	19	380	?-

FOOD	SERVING SIZE	FAT GMS	CALS	NA MGS
LONG JOHN SILVER'S® (Continued)				
Flavorbaked Chicken	1 sandwich	15	350	?-
Standard Entrees:				
Fish, Fries, Slaw, 2 Hushpuppies	2 piece dinner	48	890	1790
Fish, Fries	2 piece dinner	37	610	1480
Crispy Fish, Fries, Slaw, 2 Hushpuppies	3 piece dinner	50	980	1530
Chicken Planks, Fries, 2 Hushpuppies, Slaw	3 piece dinner	44	890	2000
Chicken Planks, Fries	2 piece dinner	26	490	1290
Clams, Fries, Slaw, 2 Hushpuppies	1 dinner	52	990	1830
Shrimp, Fries, Slaw, 2 Hushpuppies	10 piece dinner	47	840	1630
Fish (1), Chicken (1), Fries	1 dinner	32	550	1380
Fish (1), Chicken (2), Fries, Slaw, 2 Hushpuppies	1 dinner	49	950	2090
Fish (2), Shrimp (8), Fries, Slaw, 2 Hushpuppies	1 dinner	65	1140	2440
Fish (2), Shrimp (5), Chicken (1), Fries, Slaw, 2 Hushpuppies	1 dinner	65	1160	2590
Fish (2), Shrimp (4), Clams (3 oz.), Fries, Slaw, 2 Hushpuppies	1 dinner	70	1240	2630
Salads, No Dressing Or Crackers:				
Ocean Chef	1 salad	1	110	730
Seafood	1 salad	31	380	980
Standard Entrees, Kid's Meals:				
Fish (1), Fries, 1 Hushpuppy	1 dinner	28	500	1010
Fish (1), Chicken (1), Fries, 1 Hushpuppy	1 dinner	34	620	1400
Chicken Planks (2), Fries, 1 Hushpuppy	1 dinner	29	560	1310
A-La-Carte Items:				
Batter-Dipped Fish	1 piece	11	180	490
Chicken Planks	2 pieces	12	240	790
Chicken Plank	1 piece	6	120	400
Batter-Dipped Shrimp	1 piece	2	30	80
Seafood Chowder With Cod	1 serving	6	140	590
Seafood Gumbo With Cod	1 serving	8	120	740
Fries	1 serving	15	250	500
Baked Potato	1	1	160	0
Hushpuppy	1 piece	2	70	30
Corn Cobbette	1 piece	8	140	0
Green Beans	1 serving	1	40	350
Rice	1 serving	3	140	210
Cole Slaw	1 serving	6	140	260
Side Salad	1 serving	0	30	20
Roll	1	0	110	170
Desserts:				
Lemon Pie	1 piece	9	340	130
Cherry Pie	1 piece	13	360	200
Apple Pie	1 piece	13	320	420
Walnut Brownie	1 piece	22	440	150
Cookie:				
Oatmeal Raisin	1 cookie	10	160	150
Chocolate Chip	1 cookie	9	230	170
Pineapple Cream Cheesecake	1 serving	18	310	110

FOOD	SERVING SIZE	FAT GMS	CALS	NA MGS
LONG JOHN SILVER'S® (Continued)				
Condiments:				
Catsup	1 portion	0	10	140
Seafood Sauce	1 portion	0	10	180
Tartar Sauce	1 portion	5	50	40
Honey Mustard Sauce	1 portion	0	20	60
Malt Vinegar	1 portion	0	0	20
Sweet 'N Sour Sauce	1 portion	0	20	50
Ranch Dressing	1 portion	19	180	230
Creamy Italian Dressing	1 portion	3	30	280
Sea Salad Dressing	1 portion	15	140	160
Saltine Crackers	1 package	1	30	80
McDONALDS®				
Breakfast:				
Egg McMuffin	1	13	290	730
Sausage McMuffin	1	23	360	750
Sausage McMuffin With Egg	1	29	440	820
English Muffin	1	2	140	220
Sausage Biscuit	1	29	430	1130
Sausage Biscuit With Egg	1	35	520	1200
Bacon, Egg & Cheese Biscuit	1	27	450	1310
Biscuit With Biscuit Spread	1	13	260	840
Sausage	1 serving	16	170	290
Scrambled Eggs (2)	1 serving	12	170	140
Hash Brown Potatoes	1 serving	8	130	330
Hotcakes, Plain	1 serving	4	280	600
Hotcakes, Margarine (2 pats) & Syrup	1 serving	14	560	750
Cheerios	1 package	1	70	180
Wheaties	1 package	1	80	160
Apple Bran Muffin	1	1	180	210
Apple Danish	1	16	360	290
Cheese Danish	1	22	410	340
Cinnamon Raisin Danish	1	22	430	280
Raspberry Danish	1	16	400	300
Sandwiches:				
Hamburger	1	9	270	530
Cheeseburger	1	13	320	770
Quarter Pounder	1	20	420	690
With Cheese	1	29	520	1160
McLean Deluxe	1	12	340	810
With Cheese	1	16	400	1040
Big Mac	1	26	510	930
Filet-O-Fish	1	16	360	710
McGrilled Chicken Classic	1	3	250	510
McChicken	1	29	490	800
French Fries:				
Small	1 serving	10	210	140
Large	1 serving	22	450	290
Super Size	1 serving	26	540	350
Chicken McNuggets/Sauces:				
Chicken McNuggets	4 pieces	12	200	350
Chicken McNuggets	6 pieces	18	300	530
Chicken McNuggets	9 pieces	27	450	800

FOOD	SERVING SIZE	FAT GMS	CALS	NA MGS
McDONALDS® (Continued)				
Sauces:				
Hot Mustard	1 serving	4	60	250
Barbecue	1 serving	0	50	280
Sweet 'N Sour	1 serving	0	50	160
Honey	1 serving	0	50	0
Honey Mustard	1 serving	5	50	90
Salads/Dressings/Accompaniments:				
Chef Salad	1	11	210	730
Chunky Chicken Salad	1	5	160	320
Garden Salad	1	4	80	60
Side Salad	1	2	50	40
Croutons	1 serving	2	50	130
Bacon Bits	1 serving	1	20	90
Bleu Cheese Dressing	1 packet	17	190	650
Lite Vinaigrette Dressing	1 packet	2	50	240
Ranch Dressing	1 packet	21	230	550
Red French Reduced Calorie Dressing	1 packet	8	160	490
1000 Island Dressing	1 packet	13	190	510
Desserts/Milk Shakes:				
Vanilla Lowfat Yogurt Cone	1 cone	1	120	90
Lowfat Frozen Yogurt Sundaes:				
Strawberry	1	1	240	120
Hot Fudge	1	5	290	190
Hot Caramel	1	3	310	200
Nuts For Sundaes	1 serving	4	40	0
Apple Pie	1 serving	15	290	220
Cookies:				
McDonaldland	1 serving	9	260	270
Chocolaty Chip	1 serving	14	280	230
Milk Shakes, Small:				
Chocolate	16 oz.	6	350	240
Strawberry	16 oz.	5	340	170
Vanilla	16 oz.	5	310	170

OLIVE GARDEN®

FOOD	SERVING SIZE	FAT GMS	CALS	NA MGS
GARDEN FARE® Entree Selections:				
Capellini Pomodoro	1 lunch entree	8	340	530
Capellini Pomodoro	1 dinner entree	16	520	900
Capellini Primavera	1 lunch entree	5	270	650
Capellini Primavera	1 dinner entree	7	380	870
Shrimp Primavera	1 lunch entree	10	320	740
Shrimp Primavera	1 dinner entree	12	420	1060
Spaghetti & Marinara Sauce	1 lunch entree	6	340	360
Spaghetti & Marinara Sauce	1 dinner entree	9	500	530
Spaghetti & Sicilian Sauce	1 lunch entree	8	370	470
Spaghetti & Sicilian Sauce	1 dinner entree	12	530	670
Spaghetti & Tomato Sauce	1 lunch entree	7	390	1180
Spaghetti & Tomato Sauce	1 dinner entree	10	550	2290
Venetian Grilled Chicken	1 dinner entree	5	240	590
Grilled Chicken With Peppers	1 dinner entree	9	470	430
Appetizers, Breadsticks, Salad, Soup:				
Breadsticks, Plain	1 stick	2	140	270
Breadsticks, Garlic	1 stick	4	160	370
Garden Salad, No Dressing	1 order	1	70	80
House Italian Dressing	2 tablespoons	8	90	530
Minestrone Soup	6 oz.	1	80	450
House Fagioli Soup	6 oz.	5	140	300

FOOD	SERVING SIZE	FAT GMS	CALS	NA MGS

POPEYE'S® CHICKEN & BISCUITS

Chicken & Shrimp:

Mild Or Spicy Wing	1 serving	11	160	290
Mild Or Spicy Leg	1 serving	7	120	240
Mild Thigh	1 serving	23	300	620
Spicy Thigh	1 serving	23	300	450
Mild Breast	1 serving	16	270	660
Spicy Breast	1 serving	16	270	590
Nuggets	1 serving	32	410	660
Shrimp	1 serving	16	250	650

Sides and Desserts:

Biscuits	1 serving	15	250	430
Coleslaw	1 serving	11	150	270
French Fries	1 serving	12	240	610
Potatoes & Gravy	1 serving	6	100	460
Onion Rings	1 serving	19	310	210
Cajun Rice	1 serving	5	150	1260
Red Beans & Rice	1 serving	17	270	680
Corn On The Cob	1 serving	3	130	20
Apple Pie	1 serving	16	290	820

PIZZA HUT®

Pan, Medium Size:

Beef	1 slice	13	290	680
Cheese	1 slice	11	260	500
Ham	1 slice	9	240	540
Pepperoni	1 slice	12	270	570
Italian Sausage	1 slice	15	290	620
Pork Topping	1 slice	14	290	680
MEAT LOVER'S®	1 slice	18	340	840
VEGGIE LOVER'S®	1 slice	10	240	510
PEPPERONI LOVER'S®	1 slice	17	330	780
Supreme	1 slice	15	310	760
Super Supreme	1 slice	17	320	830

Hand Tossed, Medium Size:

Beef	1 slice	9	260	800
Cheese	1 slice	7	240	620
Ham	1 slice	5	210	660
Pepperoni	1 slice	8	340	690
Italian Sausage	1 slice	11	270	740
Pork Topping	1 slice	10	270	800
MEAT LOVER'S®	1 slice	11	310	960
VEGGIE LOVER'S®	1 slice	6	220	630
PEPPERONI LOVER'S®	1 slice	14	310	900
Supreme	1 slice	12	280	880
Super Supreme	1 slice	13	300	950

THIN 'N CRISPY® Pizza, Medium Size:

Beef	1 slice	11	230	710
Cheese	1 slice	8	210	530
Ham	1 slice	7	180	590
Pepperoni	1 slice	10	220	630
Italian Sausage	1 slice	12	240	650
Pork Topping	1 slice	12	240	710
MEAT LOVER'S®	1 slice	13	290	890
VEGGIE LOVER'S®	1 slice	7	190	550
PEPPERONI LOVER'S®	1 slice	16	290	860
Supreme	1 slice	13	260	800
Super Supreme	1 slice	14	270	880

Popeye's and Pizza Hut

FOOD	SERVING SIZE	FAT GMS	CALS	NA MGS
PIZZA HUT® (Continued)				
BIGFOOT™:				
Cheese	1 slice	6	190	530
Pepperoni	1 slice	7	210	590
Pepperoni, Mushroom, Italian Sausage	1 slice	8	210	670
Personal Pan Pizza:				
Pepperoni	1 pizza	28	640	1340
Supreme	1 pizza	34	720	1760
QUINCY'S®				
Breakfast:				
Escalloped Apples	1 serving	2	120	20
Bacon	1 strip	3	40	100
Corned Beef Hash	1 serving	15	210	800
Scrambled Eggs	1 serving	7	100	270
Country Ham	1 serving	6	90	1100
Oatmeal	1 serving	2	180	290
Pancakes	1 serving	3	100	250
Syrup	1 serving	0	80	0
Sausage Gravy	1 serving	6	70	150
Sausage Links	1 serving	22	230	390
Sausage Patties	1 serving	23	230	350
Steakfingers	1 serving	25	360	690
Beef Entrees:				
Chopped Steak	1 entree	34	470	100
Country Style Steak	1 entree	29	380	740
Country Steak Sandwich	1 entree	29	520	1040
Filet	1 entree	12	330	40
Prime Rib	8 oz. entree	46	570	1180
Prime Rib	16 oz. entree	93	1150	2350
Quarter Pound Hamburger	1 entree	20	410	290
Rib Eye	7.25 oz. entree	60	670	80
Rib Eye	9.5 oz. entree	78	870	100
Sirloin, Large	7.75 oz. entree	70	850	130
Sirloin, Regular	5.75 oz. entree	54	650	100
Sirloin, Petite	4 oz. entree	37	450	100
Sirloin Tips	1 entree	9	240	70
Sizzlin' Strip	1 entree	37	600	140
T-Bone	14 oz. entree	170	1610	220
Chicken Entrees:				
Grilled Chicken, Regular	4.75 oz. entree	2	130	500
Grilled Chicken, Large	9.5 oz. entree	3	250	1000
Grilled Chicken Sandwich	1 entree	5	310	810
Homestyle Chicken Filet	1 entree	24	410	1740
Grilled Trout Entree	1 entree	12	300	520
Stir-Fry Entrees:				
Beef	1 entree	77	950	590
Chicken	1 entree	66	780	1000
Rice Pilaf	1 entree	2	110	270
Soups:				
Chili With Beans	6 oz.	11	240	920
Clam Chowder	6 oz.	9	180	840
Cream of Broccoli	6 oz.	10	170	770
Vegetable Beef	6 oz.	2	90	330

FOOD	SERVING SIZE	FAT GMS	CALS	NA MGS
QUINCY'S® (Continued)				
Side Items:				
Baked Potato	1 (12 oz.)	0	370	30
Blackeyed Peas	1 serving	1	80	660
Broccoli, Plain	1 serving	1	110	30
Broccoli With Cheese Sauce	1 serving	13	250	510
Broccoli & Rice Casserole	1 serving	5	100	460
Cabbage, Steamed	1 serving	5	90	660
Candied Yams	1 serving	10	250	110
Carrots, Steamed	1 serving	4	90	90
Corn On The Cob	1 serving	1	140	540
Corn, Whole Kernel	1 serving	6	110	410
Green Beans	1 serving	1	30	190
Green Peas	1 serving	3	60	200
Hashrounds	1 serving	14	230	560
Macaroni & Cheese	1 serving	9	170	490
Mashed Potatoes	1 serving	0	70	250
Mushrooms	1 serving	12	120	360
New Potatoes	1 serving	11	190	120
Pinto Beans	1 serving	0	70	460
Refried Beans	1 serving	7	140	480
Squash	1 serving	10	110	230
Turnip Greens	1 serving	6	80	280
Vegetable Medley	1 serving	0	40	320
Breads:				
Banana Nut	1 serving	7	170	200
Biscuit	1 serving	15	270	610
Cornbread	1 serving	5	140	340
Yeast Roll	1 serving	4	160	290
Salad Dressings:				
Blue Cheese	2 tablespoons	16	160	170
French	2 tablespoons	12	130	500
Honey Mustard	2 tablespoons	6	100	220
Italian	2 tablespoons	14	140	230
Light Creamy Italian	2 tablespoons	4	70	490
Light French	2 tablespoons	4	90	290
Light Italian	2 tablespoons	2	20	490
Light 1000 Island	2 tablespoons	4	70	340
Parmesan Peppercorn	2 tablespoons	14	150	280
Ranch	2 tablespoons	11	110	200
Desserts:				
Banana Pudding	1 serving	12	240	240
Brownie Pudding Cake	1 serving	5	310	400
Chocolate Chip Cookie	1	8	60	40
Sugar Cookie	1	3	60	30
Apple Cobbler	1 serving	8	260	290
Cherry Cobbler	1 serving	8	410	190
Peach Cobbler	1 serving	8	310	190
Frozen Yogurt	1 serving	2	140	90
Hot Toppings:				
Caramel	2 tablespoons	1	110	120
Fudge	2 tablespoons	4	110	80
Pineapple	2 tablespoons	0	70	20

FOOD	SERVING SIZE	FAT GMS	CALS	NA MGS
RAX®				
"HOLD THE MAYO & OIL" MENU:				
Sandwiches, Without Mayonnaise Or Bun Oil:				
Regular Rax	1 sandwich	13	310	710
Deluxe	1 sandwich	13	330	740
Grilled Chicken	1 sandwich	7	280	930
Jr. Deluxe	1 sandwich	8	220	470
Barbecue Beef	1 sandwich	10	320	1030
Turkey	1 sandwich	4	230	1220
Cheddar Melt	1 sandwich	16	280	540
Potatoes:				
Plain	1 serving	0	210	10
With Cheese & Broccoli	1 serving	0	280	620
With Cheese	1 serving	0	270	620
With Butter	1 serving	11	310	90
With Sour Topping	1 serving	4	260	30
Soups:				
Cream of Broccoli	1 serving	4	100	510
Chicken Noodle	1 serving	1	110	300
Chili	1 serving	9	160	420
Shakes:				
Vanilla Yogurt	1 serving	1	220	140
Chocolate Yogurt	1 serving	1	310	180
Strawberry Yogurt	1 serving	0	300	150
Salads, No Dressing:				
Grilled Chicken Caesar	1 serving	5	160	1150
Caesar Side Salad	1 serving	2	40	330
Side Salad	1 serving	4	40	90
Gourmet Garden	1 serving	9	220	840
Salad Dressings:				
Fat Free Ranch	1 serving	0	30	300
Fat Free Italian	1 serving	0	10	420
Fat Free Catalina	1 serving	0	30	240
Honey French	1 serving	5	140	210
Vinaigrette	1 serving	2	30	150
Creamy Caesar	1 serving	15	140	290
RAX REGULAR MENU:				
Sandwiches, Regular Menu:				
Regular Rax	1 sandwich	22	390	710
Deluxe Rax	1 sandwich	35	520	790
Barbecue Beef	1 sandwich	20	400	1030
Barbecue Beef, Bacon & Cheddar	1 sandwich	51	720	1450
Grilled Chicken	1 sandwich	33	530	990
Jr. Deluxe	1 sandwich	25	370	510
Mushroom Melt	1 sandwich	37	600	1690
Turkey Bacon Club	1 sandwich	47	680	1900
Turkey	1 sandwich	32	480	1290
Cheddar Melt	1 sandwich	23	350	540
Philly Melt	1 sandwich	32	540	1300

Potatoes, Soups, Shakes, Salads & Most Salad Dressings On The Regular Menu Are The Same As the "Hold The Mayo & Oil" Menu

Salad Dressings:				
Buttermilk Ranch	1 serving	20	180	240
Blue Cheese	1 serving	16	150	300
1000 Island	1 serving	13	130	230

FOOD	SERVING SIZE	FAT GMS	CALS	NA MGS
SONIC®				
Hamburgers/Sandwiches:				
#1 Hamburger	1 serving	27	410	440
#2 Hamburger	1 serving	16	320	550
Cheese Added To #1/#2	1 slice	6	70	270
Bacon Cheeseburger	1 serving	39	550	840
Hickory Burger	1 serving	16	310	460
Jalapeno Burger	1 serving	41	640	1360
Super Sonic Burger & Mayo	1 serving	52	730	1020
Super Sonic Burger & Mustard	1 serving	41	640	1130
Mini Burger	1 serving	12	250	510
Mini Cheeseburger	1 serving	14	280	640
Steak Sandwich, Breaded	1 serving	42	630	1050
Chicken Sandwich, Breaded	1 serving	25	460	760
Grilled Chicken Sandwich, No Dressing	1 serving	4	220	720
Fish Sandwich	1 serving	7	280	660
B-L-T Sandwich	1 serving	19	330	600
Grilled Cheese Sandwich	1 serving	17	290	840
Coneys & Local Flavors:				
Chili Pie	1 serving	23	330	310
Regular Hot Dog	1 serving	15	260	240
Regular Cheese Coney	1 serving	23	360	340
Regular Cheese Coney & Onions	1 serving	23	360	340
Extra Long Cheese Coney	1 serving	39	640	630
Extra Long Cheese Coney With Onions	1 serving	39	640	630
Corn Dog	1 serving	15	280	700
Side Orders:				
Regular French Fries	1 serving	8	230	50
Large French Fries	1 serving	11	320	70
Large French Fries & Cheese	1 serving	20	420	470
Regular Onion Rings	1 serving	27	400	370
Large Onion Rings	1 serving	38	580	530
TATER TOTS®	1 serving	7	150	330
TATER TOTS® With Cheese	1 serving	13	220	570

SUBWAY®
Note: All Values For Sandwiches Shown Below Do Not Include Salt, Pepper, Oil, Mayo Or Salad Dressings)
Sandwiches:

Six Inch Sub:				
Veggies/Cheese/Wheat Bread	1	6	260	530
Turkey Breast/White Bread	1	8	310	1190
Four Inch Round Sandwich:				
Ham	1	7	320	670
Roast Beef	1	6	330	820
Subway Club Salad, No Dressing	1 serving	7	170	1160
Roast Turkey Breast Salad, No Dressing	1 serving	7	150	950

Sonic and Subway

FOOD	SERVING SIZE	FAT GMS	CALS	NA MGS
TACO BELL®				
BORDER LIGHTS™:				
LIGHT Taco	1	5	140	?-
LIGHT TACO SUPREME™	1	5	160	?-
LIGHT SOFT TACO SUPREME™	1	5	200	?-
LIGHT Chicken Soft Taco	1	5	180	?-
LIGHT Bean Burrito	1	6	330	?-
LIGHT Chicken Burrito	1	6	290	?-
LIGHT 7-Layer Burrito	1	9	440	?-
LIGHT BURRITO SUPREME™	1	8	350	?-
LIGHT CHICKEN BURRITO SUPREME®	1	10	410	?-
LIGHT Taco Salad:				
With Chips	1	25	680	?-
Without Chips	1	9	330	?-
Tacos And Tostadas:				
Taco	1	11	180	280
TACO SUPREME™	1	15	230	290
Soft Taco	1	12	220	540
CHICKEN TACO SUPREME®	1	15	270	550
Tostada	1	11	240	590
Chicken Soft Taco	1	10	220	550
Steak Soft Taco	1	9	220	570
Burritos:				
Bean Burrito	1	12	390	1140
Beef Burrito	1	19	430	1300
BIG BEEF BURRITO SUPREME®	1	25	530	1420
BURRITO SUPREME®	1	19	440	1180
Chicken Burrito	1	13	350	850
CHICKEN BURRITO SUPREME®	1	23	520	1130
Chili Cheese Burrito	1	18	390	980
Combo Burrito	1	16	410	1220
7 Layer Burrito	1	21	490	1120
STEAK BURRITO SUPREME®	1	23	500	1350
Specialty Items:				
NACHOS BELL GRANDE®	1 serving	34	630	950
Nachos Supreme	1 serving	18	360	470
Nachos	1 serving	18	350	400
BEEF MEXIMELT®	1 serving	14	260	710
Mexican Pizza	1 serving	38	570	1000
Pintos 'N Cheese	1 serving	9	190	640
Taco Salad	1 serving	55	840	1130
Cinnamon Twists	1 serving	6	140	190
Side Orders And Condiments:				
Hot Taco Sauce	1 serving	0	0	90
Mild Taco Sauce	1 serving	0	0	10
Picante Sauce	1 serving	0	0	130
Salsa	1 serving	0	30	710
Pico De Gallo	1 serving	0	10	70
Sour Cream	1 serving	4	40	10
Guacamole	1 serving	3	40	130
Ranch Dressing	1 serving	14	140	330
Nacho Cheese Sauce	1 serving	4	50	200
Red Sauce	1 serving	0	10	260
Green Sauce	1 serving	0	0	140

FOOD	SERVING SIZE	FAT GMS	CALS	NA MGS
"TCBY"®				
Soft-Serve Frozen Yogurt:				
No Sugar Added & Nonfat	1/2 cup	0	80	40
Nonfat	1/2 cup	0	110	60
Regular	1/2 cup	3	130	60
Sorbet	1/2 cup	0	100	30
TGI FRIDAY'S®				
LITE MENU:				
Friday's GARDENBURGER® Sandwich	1 serving	8	390	?-
Chili Yogurt Sauce	1 serving	0	40	?-
Blackeyed Pea & Corn Salsa	1 serving	2	170	?-
Pacific Coast Tuna With Fresh Vegetables Over Linguini, No Dressing	1 serving	7	280	?-
Pacific Coast Chicken With Fresh Vegetables Over Linguini, No Dressing	1 serving	13	320	?-
Oriental Vinaigrette Dressing	1 serving	12	160	?-
Garden Dagwood Sandwich	1 serving	13	390	?-
WENDY'S®				
Sandwiches:				
Hamburger:				
Plain Single	1	15	350	510
Single With Everything	1	23	440	860
Big Bacon Classic	1	36	640	1500
Junior	1	9	270	600
Junior Cheeseburger	1	13	320	770
Junior Bacon Cheeseburger	1	25	440	870
Junior Cheeseburger Deluxe	1	20	390	820
Chicken Sandwich:				
Grilled	1	7	290	720
Breaded	1	20	450	740
Club	1	25	520	990
Junior Or Kid's Meal:				
Hamburger Meal	1	9	270	600
Cheeseburger Meal	1	13	310	770
French Fries:				
Small	1 serving	12	240	150
Medium	1 serving	17	340	210
Biggie	1 serving	20	420	260
Baked Potato:				
Plain	1 serving	0	310	30
Bacon & Cheese	1 serving	18	530	1280
Broccoli & Cheese	1 serving	14	460	440
Cheese	1 serving	23	560	610
Chili & Cheese	1 serving	24	610	700
Sour Cream & Chives	1 serving	6	380	40
Sour Cream	1 packet	6	60	20
Whipped Margarine	1 packet	5	60	110
Chili & Accompaniments:				
Small	8 ounces	6	190	670
Large	12 ounces	9	290	1000
Cheddar Cheese, Shredded	2 tablespoons	6	70	110
Saltine Crackers	2 crackers	1	30	80

FOOD	SERVING SIZE	FAT GMS	CALS	NA MGS
WENDY'S® (Continued)				
Chicken Nuggets	1 serving (6)	20	280	600
Sauces:				
Barbecue	1 packet	0	50	100
Honey	1 packet	0	50	0
Sweet & Sour	1 packet	0	50	60
Sweet Mustard	1 packet	1	50	140
Garden Spot Salad Bar:				
Applesauce	2 tablespoons	0	30	0
Bacon Bits	2 tablespoons	2	40	540
Broccoli	1/4 cup	0	0	0
Cantaloupe, Sliced	2 pieces	0	30	0
Carrots	1/4 cup	0	10	10
Cauliflower	1/4 cup	0	0	0
Cheddar Chips	2 tablespoons	4	70	200
Cheese, Shredded, Imitation	2 tablespoons	4	50	230
Chicken Salad	2 tablespoons	5	70	140
Chives	1 tablespoon	0	0	0
Chow Mein Noodles	1/4 cup	2	40	30
Cole Slaw	2 tablespoons	3	50	70
Cottage Cheese	2 tablespoons	2	30	130
Croutons	2 tablespoons	1	30	80
Cucumbers	2 slices	0	0	0
Eggs, Hard Cooked	2 tablespoons	3	40	30
Green Peas	2 tablespoons	0	20	30
Green Peppers	2 pieces	0	0	0
Honeydew Melon	2 slices	0	40	20
Jalapeno Peppers	1 tablespoon	0	0	160
Lettuce	1 cup	0	10	10
Mushrooms	1/4 cup	0	0	0
Olives, Black	2 tablespoons	2	20	120
Orange, Sectioned	2 pieces	0	20	0
Pasta Salad	2 tablespoons	0	30	80
Peaches, Sliced	1 piece	0	20	0
Pepperoni, Sliced	6 pieces	3	30	70
Pineapple, Chunked	4 pieces	0	20	0
Potato Salad	2 tablespoons	7	80	180
Pudding, Chocolate	1/4 cup	0	70	60
Pudding, Vanilla	1/4 cup	0	70	60
Red Onions	3 rings	0	0	0
Seafood Salad	1/4 cup	4	70	300
Sesame Bread Stick	1 stick	0	20	20
Strawberries	4	0	40	0
Strawberry Banana Dessert	1/4 cup	0	30	0
Sunflower Seeds And Raisins	2 tablespoons	5	80	0
Tomato Wedges	6 pieces	0	30	0
Turkey Ham, Diced	2 tablespoons	4	50	280
Watermelon Wedges	1 piece	0	20	0
Salad/SuperBar:				
Salad Dressings:				
Blue Cheese	2 tablespoons (1 ladle)	19	180	180
Celery Seed	2 tablespoons	7	100	220
French	2 tablespoons	11	120	300
French, Fat Free	2 tablespoons	0	40	180
French, Sweet Red	2 tablespoons	10	130	250
Hidden Valley Ranch	2 tablespoons	10	90	210

Wendy's

FOOD	SERVING SIZE	FAT GMS	CALS	NA MGS
WENDY'S® (Continued)				
Salad Dressings (Continued):				
Hidden Valley Ranch, Reduced Calorie	2 tablespoons	5	60	280
Italian Caesar	2 tablespoons	16	150	230
Italian, Golden	2 tablespoons	7	90	450
Italian, Reduced Calorie	2 tablespoons	3	40	330
Salad Oil	1 tablespoon	14	130	0
Thousand Island	2 tablespoons	13	130	160
Wine Vinegar	1 tablespoon	0	0	0
Fresh Salads To Go/No Dressing:				
Caesar Side	1 serving	5	110	580
Deluxe Garden	1 serving	6	110	320
Grilled Chicken	1 serving	8	200	690
Side	1 serving	3	60	160
Taco	1 serving	30	580	1060
Breadstick, Soft	1 each	3	130	250
Super Bar (Where Available):				
Alfredo Sauce	1/4 cup	2	30	250
Cheese Sauce	1/4 cup	1	30	190
Macaroni & Cheese	1/2 cup	6	130	320
Parmesan Cheese, Grated	2 tablespoons	5	70	220
Picante Sauce	2 tablespoons	0	10	260
Refried Beans	1/4 cup	3	80	300
Rice, Spanish	1/4 cup	1	60	390
Rotini	1/2 cup	2	90	?-
Sour Topping	2 tablespoons	5	60	30
Spaghetti Sauce	1/4 cup	0	30	340
Spaghetti Meat Sauce	1/4 cup	2	50	230
Taco Chips	8 chips	7	120	90
Taco Meat	2 tablespoons	4	80	200
Taco Sauce	2 tablespoons	0	10	110
Taco Shells	1	4	60	20
Tortilla, Flour	1	3	110	210
Frosty Dairy Dessert:				
Small	12 oz.	10	340	200
Medium	16 oz.	13	460	260
Large	20 oz.	17	570	330
Chocolate Chip Cookie	1	11	270	150

Wendy's

Chapter 16

HOW DO YOU ALTER RECIPES FOR LOWER FAT CONTENT?
PLUS SAMPLE RECIPES

Our clients often bring in their favorite recipes for help in altering them to lower the fat content. We thought you, too, might like to see how to lower fat in a full fat recipe to more healthful levels. The recipes in this chapter are some of our favorites. We include the original recipe with its fat, calorie and sodium content and, next to it, the lower fat version. Compare the lower fat version's fat and calorie content to the higher values shown for the original. Gayle Lopes, R.D., L.D., of NCES, Inc. calculated the nutritional values using NUTRITIONIST IV, a computer nutritional analysis program.

If you decide to lower fat content in some of your favorite recipes, use the information in the TABLE OF FOOD VALUES. For the person who enjoys working with his/her computer, there are several inexpensive nutritional analyses programs on the market. Check with your local software store.

GENERAL HINTS

There are several ways you can lower fat in a recipe. You can leave an ingredient out. You can replace part of a high fat ingredient with a low or nonfat ingredient. You can also replace all of a high fat ingredient with a low or nonfat ingredient. We will use all of these techniques in the recipes to follow.

Many recipes list a large amount of fat for use in sautéing onions, etc. or for browning meat. This amount of fat can be lowered substantially or cut out altogether without altering the taste of the product significantly. Spray your pan with a non-stick pan spray and leave out this fat altogether.

In one of our earlier chapters, we had a list of lower fat alternatives to try instead of the regular item—e.g., lower fat cheeses rather than full fat cheeses. You may wish to consult this list before modifying your own recipes.

When baking or broiling, try spraying the food with a non stick pan spray to help keep it moist. Bake fish, other protein foods or vegetables on a sprayed pan. Then spray the top side of the item before adding herb and spice seasonings.

For grilling, try an oil free marinade but remember to spray your grill with the non-stick pan spray. Making or purchasing a good herb or spice blend can save time and help you turn out delicious foods. Included are two recipes for blends we find to be quite tasty. Recipes begin on the next page.

Abbreviations used: T = tablespoon; t = teaspoon; c = cup; chpd = chopped; oz = ounce; approx = approximately; F = Fahrenheit; mgs = milligrams; gms = grams; cal = calorie; lb = pounds; svg = serving

SOUR CREAM MUFFINS

Original Version (12 muffins)	Lower Fat Version (12 muffins)
1 egg, beaten	1 egg, beaten
1 c. sour cream	1 c. plain nonfat yogurt
2 T. melted margarine	2 T. melted margarine
2 c. sifted all-purpose flour	2 c. sifted all-purpose flour
1/4 c. sugar	1/4 c. sugar
2 t. baking powder	2 t. baking powder
1/2 t. baking soda	1/2 t. baking soda
1/2 t. salt	1/2 t. salt
1/4 c. whole milk	1/4 c. skim milk
1. Preheat oven to 400 degrees F. 2. Beat egg and sour cream until light. 3. Add rest of ingredients. Stir only until dry ingredients are moistened. Do not overmix. 4. Fill twelve 2 3/4" muffin cups half full with the batter. Bake in oven about 20 minutes.	1. Same. 2. Beat egg and yogurt together. 3. Same. 4. Same.
Per Svg Fat Gms 7 Calories 160 Sodium Mgs 240	**Per Svg** 3 130 250

SOUR CREAM CORN BREAD

Original Version (8 servings)	Lower Fat Version (8 servings)
3/4 c. yellow corn meal	3/4 c. yellow corn meal
1 c. unsifted all-purpose flour	1 c. unsifted all-purpose flour
1/4 c. sugar	1/4 c. sugar
2 t. baking powder	2 t. baking powder
1/2 t. baking soda	1/2 t. baking soda
1/2 t. salt	1/2 t. salt
1 c. sour cream	1 c. plain nonfat yogurt
1/4 c. whole milk	1/4 c. skim milk
1 egg, beaten	1 egg, beaten
2 T. vegetable oil	2 T. vegetable oil
1. Preheat oven to 425 degrees F. 2. Stir all ingredients together just enough to blend. Do not overmix. 3. Pour into 8" square greased pan and bake about 20 minutes.	1. Same. 2. Same. 3. Spray an 8" square pan with non stick pan spray. Pour into pan and bake about 20minutes.
Per Svg Fat Gms 11 Calories 240 Sodium Mgs 330	**Per Svg** 5 190 340

VEGETABLE AND OLIVE SALAD

Original Version (Serves 6)	Lower Fat Version (Serves 6)
1 head of butterhead lettuce, torn	1 head of butterhead lettuce, torn
36 pitted ripe olives	18 pitted ripe olives
1 head of romaine lettuce, torn	1 head of romaine lettuce, torn
1 c. radishes, sliced	1 c. radishes, sliced
2 carrots, grated	2 carrots, grated
1 c. celery, sliced	1 c. celery, sliced
1 c. plain nonfat yogurt	1 c. plain nonfat yogurt
1 T. Dijon mustard	1 T. Dijon mustard
1/4 t. salt	1/4 t. salt
1/4 t. pepper	1/4 t. pepper
1. Mix lettuces, olives, radishes, carrots, and celery together in large bowl.	1. Same.
2. Combine yogurt, mustard, salt, and pepper. Add to greens and toss well.	2. Same.

	Per Svg		Per Svg
Fat Gms	3		2
Calories	90		70
Sodium Mgs	450		330

CHILI

Original Version (4 servings)	Lower Fat Version (8 servings)
1 pound lean ground beef	1/2 pound extra lean ground beef
1 large onion, chpd	1 large onion, chpd
2 garlic cloves, chpd	2 garlic cloves, chpd
3 T. olive oil	1 t. olive oil
3 c. water	3 c. water or more to taste
	1 c. tomato paste, unsalted
1 1/3 c. canned tomatoes, chpd	1 (28 oz.) can tomatoes, chpd
1 green pepper, seeded, chpd	1 green pepper, seeded, chpd
2 T. chili powder or more	2 T. chili powder or more
1/2 t. salt	(Salt omitted)
1 t. whole cumin seed	1 t. whole cumin seed
1/2 t. ground cumin seed	1/2 t. ground cumin seed
1/2 t. celery seed	1/2 t. celery seed
1/4 t. cayenne pepper	1/4 t. cayenne pepper
1/8 t. basil, crushed	1/8 t. basil, crushed
1 small bay leaf	1 small bay leaf
1 can (1 lb.) kidney beans (approx. 1 1/2 cups)	4 1/2 cups cooked kidney beans, unsalted (cooked from scratch)

(See next page for directions and nutrient analyses.)

CHILI (Continued)

1. Sauté onion and garlic in oil until golden.	1. Sauté onion and garlic in oil until golden.
2. Brown ground beef in separate Drain well.	2. Brown ground beef in skillet. separate skillet. Drain well.
3. Transfer above ingredients to sauce pan.	3. Transfer above ingredients to large soup pan.
4. Add rest of ingredients.	4. Add rest of ingredients.
5. Simmer uncovered for 2-3 hours.	5. Simmer uncovered for 2-3 hours.

	Per Svg		Per Svg
Fat Gms	23		5
Calories	460		350
Sodium Mgs	860		730

Note: The Lower Fat Version makes twice as many servings as the Original Version.

WHITE CLAM SAUCE WITH SPAGHETTI

Original Version (4 servings)
1 (10 oz.) can minced clams
(6 oz. clams without juice)
1 clove minced garlic
3 T. olive oil
1/4 t. thyme
1/4 t. pepper
1/4 c. parsley, chpd
1/2 c. Parmesan cheese

6 c. cooked spaghetti,
(no oil or salt added)

Lower Fat Version (4 servings)
1 (10 oz.) can minced clams
(6 oz. clams without juice)
1 clove minced garlic
No oil
1/4 t. thyme
1/4 t. pepper
1/4 cup parsley, chpd
1/2 c. Parmesan cheese

6 c. cooked spaghetti,
(no oil or salt added)

1. Sauté garlic in oil.	1. Simmer garlic in small amount of juice from canned clams.
2. Heat clams in juice from can. Add garlic, thyme and pepper.	2. Add clams and rest of juice to garlic. Add thyme, and pepper. Heat.
3. Add clam mixture, parsley, and Parmesan cheese to spaghetti. Serve.	3. Same.

	Per Svg		Per Svg
Fat Gms	16		6
Calories	480		390
Sodium Mgs	270		270

SALMON LOAF

Original Version (8 servings)
1 can salmon, (approx. 1 lb.) drained

1 c. (2 slices) soft bread crumbs
1/4 c. margarine, melted
2 eggs, beaten
1 1/2 T. onion, minced
2 t. parsley, minced
1 T. green pepper, minced
1/4 t. Worcestershire sauce
Dash of Tabasco sauce

Lower Fat Version (8 servings)
1 can salmon, (approx. 1 lb.) drained
1 c. (2 slices) soft bread crumbs
(Leave out margarine)
1 egg, plus 2 egg whites, beaten
1 1/2 T. onion, minced
2 t. parsley, minced
1 T. green pepper, minced
1/4 t. Worcestershire sauce
Dash of Tabasco sauce

1. Preheat oven to 350 degrees F. 2. Grease a loaf pan. 3. Mix all ingredients together. 4. Press mixture into pan. 5. Bake for about 35-40 minutes.	1. Same. 2. Spray a loaf pan with non stick pan spray. 3. Same. 4. Same. 5. Same.

	Per Svg		Per Svg
Fat Gms	11		4
Calories	160		100
Sodium Mgs	370		310

SPINACH RICOTTA CHEESE TART

Original Version (8 servings)
1 prebaked pie shell
2 packages (10-oz.) frozen chpd spinach
1/4 c. onion, diced
1/4 c. margarine
1/4 t. ground nutmeg
Dash pepper
1 (15-oz.) carton ricotta cheese, part skim milk (approx. 2 cups)
1 c. half and half
1/2 c. grated Parmesan cheese
3 eggs, beaten slightly

Lower Fat Version (6 servings)
No pie shell
2 packages (10-oz.) frozen chpd spinach
1/4 c. onion, diced
1 t. margarine
1/4 t. ground nutmeg
Dash pepper
1 (15-oz.) carton ricotta cheese, part skim milk (approx. 2 cups)
1 c. skim milk
1/2 c. grated Parmesan cheese
3 eggs, beaten slightly

1. Cook spinach according to package directions. 2. Drain well and set aside. Sauté onion in margarine in skillet. Add spinach, nutmeg, and pepper. 3. Combine ricotta cheese, half and half, Parmesan cheese, and eggs in bowl, mixing thoroughly. Stir in spinach mixture.	1. Same. 2. Same. 3. Same, except use skim milk instead of half and half.

(See next page for remainder of directions and nutrient analyses.)

SPINACH RICOTTA CHEESE TART (Continued)

4. Pour into prebaked pie shell and bake at 350 degrees F. for about 50 minutes or until set and lightly browned.	4. Pour mixture into pan. Spray pan with non stick spray and bake for about 50 minutes or until set and lightly browned.

	Per Svg		Per Svg
Fat Gms	23		9
Calories	330		180
Sodium Mgs	460		300

CHICKEN STROGANOFF

Original Version (4 servings)	Lower Fat Version (4 servings)
1 medium onion, chpd	1 medium onion, chpd
1/4 c. olive oil	1 t. olive oil
1/2 lb. mushrooms, sliced	1/2 lb. mushrooms, sliced
1 T. flour	1 T. flour
2 t. paprika	2 t. paprika
1/4 t. salt	1/4 t. salt
1/4 t. basil	1/4 t. basil
1/4 t. thyme	1/4 t. thyme
1/2 c. chicken broth, canned	1/2 c. chicken broth, canned
1/2 c. dry vermouth	1/2 c. dry vermouth
1/2 c. sour cream	1/2 c. nonfat plain yogurt
2 c. cooked chicken, skinless, diced	2 c. cooked chicken, skinless, diced
2 t. lemon juice	2 t. lemon juice
1 t. dill weed	1 t. dill weed

1. Sauté onion in oil until golden.	1. Same.
2. Add mushrooms. Cook and stir 3 to 5 minutes longer. Blend in flour, paprika, salt, basil, and thyme. Cook 1 minute. Remove from heat.	2. Same.
3. Stir in chicken broth and wine. Return to heat. Cook, stirring constantly until mixture thickens. Cover. Simmer 5 minutes.	3. Same.
4. Remove from heat. Blend in sour cream, chicken, lemon juice, and dill. Heat thoroughly, but do not allow to boil.	4. Remove from heat. Blend in yogurt, chicken, lemon juice, and dill. Heat thoroughly, but do not allow to boil.
5. Serve over hot cooked noodles. (Not included in calculations below.)	5. Same.

	Per Svg		Per Svg
Fat Gms	29		10
Calories	420		270
Sodium Mgs	310		310

MEATLOAF

Original Version (10 servings)
2 c. (4 slices) soft bread crumbs
1 c. chopped onion
2 eggs, beaten
2 pounds lean ground beef
2 T. Worcestershire Sauce
1 1/2 t. dry mustard
1/2 t. salt
1/2 t. freshly ground pepper
3/4 c. whole milk

Lower Fat Version (10 servings)
2 c. (4 slices) soft bread crumbs
1 c. chopped onion
1 egg, plus 2 egg whites, beaten
2 pounds extra lean ground beef
2 T. Worcestershire Sauce
1 1/2 t. dry mustard
1/2 t. salt
1/2 t. freshly ground pepper
3/4 c. skim milk

1. Preheat oven to 350 degrees F. 2. Mix all ingredients together in a large bowl. 3. Grease a loaf pan. 4. Press mixture into pan. 5. Bake for 45 minutes.	1. Same. 2. Same. 3. Spray a loaf pan with non stick spray. 4. Same. 5. Same.

	Per Svg		Per Svg
Fat Gms	21		16
Calories	300		260
Sodium Mgs	280		280

PRETZEL OVEN-FRIED CHICKEN

Original Version (6 servings)
6 chicken breast halves
1 c. sour cream
1 T. lemon juice
1 t. Worcestershire sauce
1/2 t. salt
1/4 t. pepper
4 oz. crushed pretzels

Lower Fat Version (6 servings)
6 chicken breast halves
1 c. plain nonfat yogurt
1 T. lemon juice
1 t. Worcestershire sauce
(Omit salt)
1/4 t. pepper
4 oz. crushed pretzels

1. Preheat oven to 350 degrees F. 2. Mix sour cream, lemon juice, Worcestershire sauce, salt, and pepper. 3. Dip the chicken pieces in the mixture and coat well. 4. Roll them in the crushed pretzels. 5. Place the chicken pieces in a greased pan and bake for about 50 minutes or until crisp and brown.	1. Same. 2. Mix yogurt, lemon juice, Worcestershire sauce and pepper. 3. Same. 4. Same. 5. Place the chicken pieces in a pan sprayed with non stick pan spray. Rest same.

	Per Svg		Per Svg
Fat Gms	17		4
Calories	350		240
Sodium Mgs	590		420

ROAST PORK

We are presenting only one version here because this recipe contains no ingredients, except the pork, which contains fat. (10 servings)

2 1/2 pounds pork loin strip, trimmed of all visible fat
1 green onion, chpd
1 clove garlic, chpd
1 T. picante sauce
2 T. sherry
2 T. soy sauce
1 t. brown sugar
1/4 t. salt
1/4 t. paprika

1. Place pork in a glass pan. Mix rest of ingredients and coat pork with the mixture. Leave overnight in the refrigerator. Turn over once or twice.
2. Remove from marinade. Roast in preheated oven for 40 minutes per pound. Baste with marinade during baking.
3. Remove from oven. Cool and slice thin. Serve at room temperature.

	Per Svg
Fat Gms	7
Calories	170
Sodium Mgs	340

BAKED ORANGE ROUGHY

Original Version (4 servings)	Lower Fat Version (4 servings)
1 pound orange roughy	1 pound orange roughy
2 T. olive oil	Pan spray
Garlic powder	Garlic powder
Onion powder	Onion powder
Paprika	Paprika
Dill weed	Dill weed
1/2 t. salt	(Omit salt)
Pepper	Pepper

Original	Lower Fat
1. Preheat oven to 400 degrees F.	1. Same.
2. Coat fish with oil.	2. Spray pan and fish with non stick pan spray.
3. Sprinkle rest of ingredients to taste on fish.	3. Same.
4. Bake for approx. 15 minutes in oven.	4. Same.

	Per Svg	Per Svg
Fat Gms	8	1
Calories	140	80
Sodium Mgs	350	80

SOUR CREAM POTATO SALAD

Original Version (6 servings)	**Lower Fat Version (6 servings)**
6 c. cooked potatoes, diced	6 c. cooked potatoes, diced
1/4 c. onion, chpd	1/4 c. onion, chpd
1/4 c. celery, chpd	1/4 c. celery, chpd
1/2 c. parsley, minced	1/2 c. parsley, minced
1 t. celery seed	1 t. celery seed
1/2 t. salt	(Omit salt)
1/2 t. pepper	1/2 t. pepper
4 eggs, hard boiled	2 eggs, hard boiled
1 c. sour cream	1 c. plain nonfat yogurt
1/2 c. mayonnaise	1/2 c. fat free salad dressing, mayonnaise type
1/4 c. vinegar	1/4 c. vinegar
1 t. prepared mustard	1 t. prepared mustard
3/4 c. pared cucumber, diced	3/4 c. pared cucumber, diced
1. Mix potatoes, onion, celery, parsley, celery seed, salt, pepper, and eggs in large bowl.	1. Same.
2. Combine sour cream, mayonnaise, vinegar, and mustard.	2. Combine yogurt, salad dressdressing, vinegar, mustard.
3. Pour over potato mixture and mix well. Add cucumber just before serving.	3. Same.

	Per Svg		Per Svg
Fat Gms	28		2
Calories	490		300
Sodium Mgs	360		360

SPICE BLENDS (ALSO SALT FREE)

CAJUN SPICE BLEND
(Makes about 1/2 cup)
1/4 cup paprika
1 T. ground hot red pepper
1 T. ground white pepper
1 T. ground black pepper
1 T. onion powder
1 T. garlic powder
2 t. oregano
1 t. thyme

CURRY BLEND
(Makes about 1/2 cup)
1 T. turmeric
1 T. coriander
1 T. cumin
1 T. garlic powder
1 T. ground ginger
1 T. ground cardamom seed
1 t. celery seed
1 t. ground black pepper
1 t. mustard powder
1 t. red pepper
1 t. ground ginger

Note: Fat, calorie, and sodium free.

ZUCCHINI IN FOIL

Original Version (4 servings)	Lower Fat Version (4 servings)
4 medium zucchini squash 1/4 cup olive oil Garlic powder Dill weed Herb blend	4 medium zucchini squash Pan spray Garlic powder Dill weed Herb blend
1. Place zucchini on squares of aluminum foil. Add 1 T. oil to each squash. Sprinkle to taste with other ingredients. 2. Wrap foil around squash and grill over a hot grill for approx. 30 minutes.	1. Place zucchini on squares of aluminum foil. Spray each squash with non stick pan spray. Sprinkle to taste with other ingredients. 2. Same.

	Per Svg		Per Svg
Fat Gms	14		0
Calories	140		20
Sodium Mgs	5		5

SALMON DIP

Original Version (16 servings– approx. 3 T. each)	Lower Fat Version (16 servings– approx. 3 T. each)
1 can (approx. 1 lb.) salmon 1 (8 oz.) pkg. cream cheese 1 T. lemon juice 1 t. prepared horseradish 1/2 c. pecans, chpd 3 T. parsley, minced 2 t. onion, minced	1 can (approx. 1 lb.) salmon 1 (8 oz.) pkg. fat free cream cheese 1 T. lemon juice 1 t. prepared horseradish 1/4 c. pecans, chpd 3 T. parsley, minced 2 t. onion, minced
1. Drain salmon, break up 2. Combine all ingredients. Mix thoroughly. 3. Chill for several hours before serving. 4. Serve with assorted crackers.	1. Same. 2. Same. 3. Same. 4. Same.

	Per Svg		Per Svg
Fat Gms	9		3
Calories	110		60
Sodium Mgs	170		210

APPENDIX A
METROPOLITAN HEIGHT/WEIGHT TABLES

The Metropolitan Life Foundation provided these guidelines in 1959 and 1983. Weights in the 1983 version were based on the lowest death rates for men and women at ages 25 to 59 for various heights and body frame sizes.

The first table below assists you in determining your frame size and the second table is the 1983 Metropolitan Height and Weight table.

Both tables are provided courtesy of the Metropolitan Life Insurance Company.

TO MAKE AN APPROXIMATION OF YOUR FRAME SIZE...

Extend your arm and bend the forearm upward at a 90 degree angle. Keep fingers straight and turn the inside of your wrist toward your body. If you have a caliper, use it to measure the space between the two prominent bones on **either** side of your elbows. Without a caliper, place thumb and index finger of your other hand on these two bones. Measure the space between your fingers against a ruler or tape measure. Compare it with these tables that list elbow measurements for **medium-framed** men and women. Measurements lower than those listed indicate you have a small frame. Higher measurements indicate a large frame.

Height in 1" Heels MEN	Elbow Breadth	Height in 1" Heels WOMEN	Elbow Breadth
5'2"—5'3"	2 1/2"—2 7/8"	4'10"—4'11"	2 1/4"—2 1/2"
5'4"—5'7"	2 5/8"—2 7/8"	5'0"—5'3"	2 1/4"—2 1/2"
5'8"—5'11"	2 3/4"—3"	5'4"—5'7"	2 3/8"—2 5/8"
6'0"—6'3"	2 3/4"—3 1/8"	5'8"—5'11"	2 3/8"—2 5/8"
6'4"	2 7/8"—3 1/4"	6'0"	2 1/2"—2 3/4"

1983 METROPOLITAN HEIGHT AND WEIGHT TABLES

The weights on the tables are representative of adults (between the ages of 25-59), based on lowest mortality (death rates). The weight is in pounds according to frame size in indoor clothing weighing 5 pounds for men and 3 pounds for women; height includes shoes with 1" heels.

Height Inches	MEN Small Frame	MEN Medium Frame	MEN Large Frame	WOMEN Small Frame	WOMEN Medium Frame	WOMEN Large Frame
58				102–111	109–121	118–131
59				103–113	111–123	120–134
60				104–115	113–126	122–137
61				106–118	115–129	125–140
62	128–134	131–141	138–150	108–121	118–132	128–143
63	130–136	133–143	140–153	111–124	121–135	131–147
64	132–138	135–145	142–156	114–127	124–138	134–151
65	134–140	137–148	144–160	117–130	127–141	137–155
66	136–142	139–151	146–164	120–133	130–144	140–159
67	138–145	142–154	149–168	123–136	133–147	143–163
68	140–148	145–157	152–172	126–139	136–150	146–167
69	142–151	148–160	155–176	129–142	139–153	149–170
70	144–154	151–163	158–180	132–145	142–156	152–173
71	146–157	154–166	161–184	135–148	145–159	155–176
72	149–160	157–170	164–188	138–151	148–162	158–179
73	152–164	160–174	168–192			
74	155–168	164–178	172–197			
75	158–172	167–182	176–202			
76	162–176	171–187	181–207			